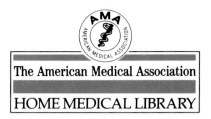

The American Medical Association

HOME MEDICAL LIBRARY

DIET AND NUTRITION

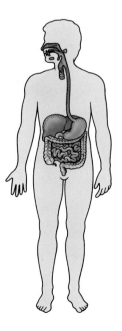

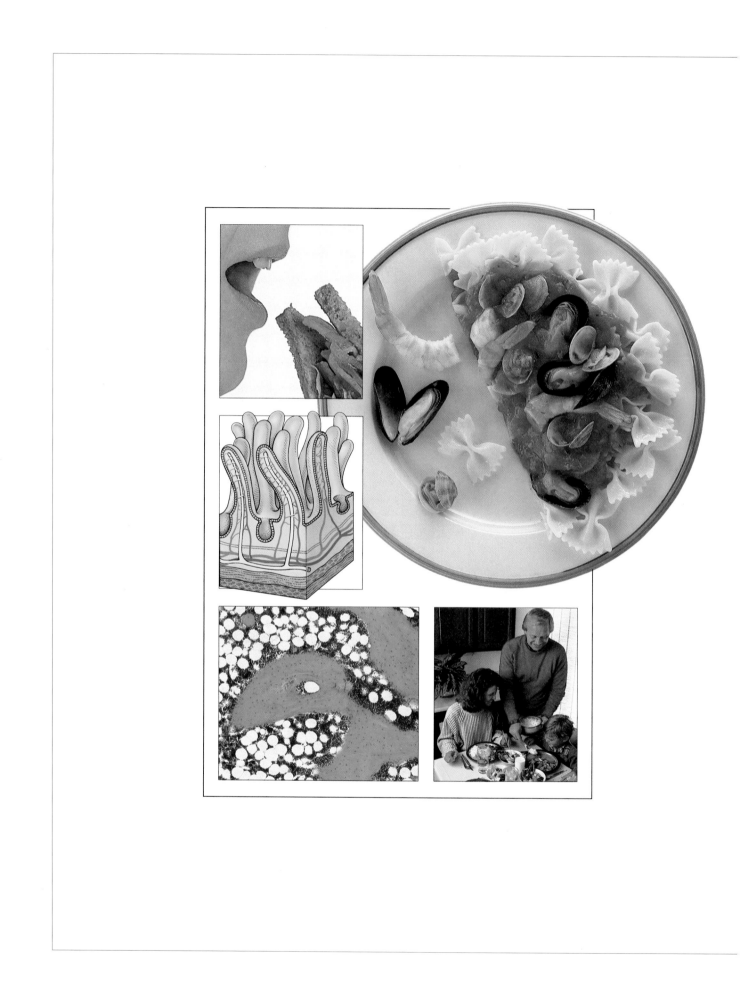

THE AMERICAN MEDICAL ASSOCIATION

DIET AND NUTRITION

Medical Editor
CHARLES B. CLAYMAN, MD

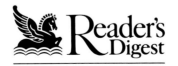

THE READER'S DIGEST ASSOCIATION, INC.
Pleasantville, New York/Montreal

Library of Congress Cataloging in Publication Data

Diet and nutrition medical editor, Charles B. Clayman.
          p.   cm — (American Medical Association home medical library)
          At head of title: The American Medical Association.
          ISBN 0-89577-358-9
          1. Nutrition — Popular works. 2. Nutritionally induced diseases —
Popular works. 3. Nutrition disorders — Popular works.
I. Clayman, Charles B. II. American Medical Association.
III. Series.
QP141.D493 1991
813.2 — dc20
                                                        90-8382
                                                        CIP

FOREWORD

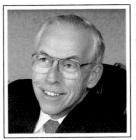

Most Americans have come to believe that good health is not a matter of luck, but rather something that we can do something about. We have also come to understand that our environment and our life-styles – including the food we eat – have a major influence on good health. Our eating patterns are one of the factors over which we have the most control. Recognizing this, many physicians try to spend more time discussing the nutritional concerns of patients and their families. This volume of the AMA Home Medical Library offers specific information on the vital link between food and health.

Today's health-conscious consumer eagerly asks pointed questions about the role of nutrition in maintaining health and preventing disease. The 1988 Surgeon General's Report on Nutrition and Health calls attention to a major shift over the years in the way in which dietary patterns affect our health – a shift away from nutrient deficiencies as problems toward one of dietary excesses and obesity. The report also underscores the pervasive influence of dietary patterns on the quality of our lives, beginning with the health of pregnant women and their infants and ranging through dietary factors associated with aging.

Most Americans are concerned about controlling their weight and staying physically fit. At the same time, economic and social changes, along with improvements in our food supply, have transformed our food choices well as our eating behaviors. In that connection, we hope that you and your family will be able to make regular use of the advice on diet, exercise, and life-styles contained in this volume.

Food and our choices of what we eat continue to be integral parts of life and a natural expression of conviviality. In recognition of that situation, we at the American Medical Association wish you and your family the best of health.

James S. Todd, MD

JAMES S. TODD, MD
Executive Vice President
American Medical Association

CONTENTS

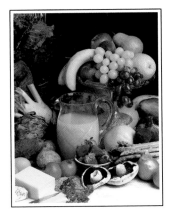

CHAPTER ONE

THE IMPORTANCE OF DIET

INTRODUCTION

WORLD DIETS AND HEALTH

ARE YOU ON THE RIGHT PATH TO A HEALTHY DIET?

EVERY YEAR, millions of American tourists and travelers visit all corners of the world. Apart from geographical differences, the most obvious variations are seen in the races, clothing, foods, traditions, and social organization of the people. One thing the traveler is unlikely to see, however, is how the pattern of health and disease in distant countries varies from that of the US. The populations of many developing countries suffer from diseases associated with poverty (such as tuberculosis) or inadequate sanitation and poor environmental quality (such as cholera), as well as a variety of nutritional deficiencies. But even affluent communities in countries` such as Japan and in southern Europe have causes of sickness that are different than those seen in the US. As explained in WORLD

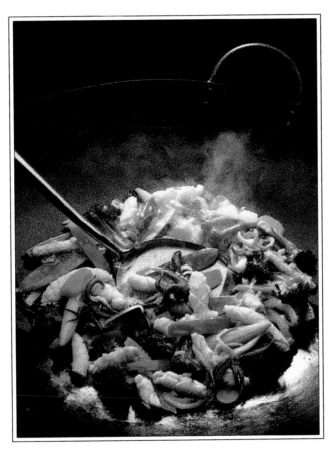

DIETS AND HEALTH – the first section of this chapter – by comparing the dietary habits and the predominant causes of death in many regions, theoretical links can be suggested between diet and diseases ranging from coronary heart disease and hypertension to certain types of cancer. These links are of enormous interest today, both to consumers and to doctors, and form the basis for continuing research.

The food that is available and the diet eaten by the people in each country or culture has advantages and disadvantages. In the US and other developed countries, the availability of a wide range of inexpensive, wholesome, and fortified foods has greatly diminished the disorders caused by vitamin or mineral deficiencies. However, ironically, those problems have been replaced by the diseases of an affluent life-style – disorders that are associated with (though not necessarily caused by) a high intake of fat, sugar, and total calories, not enough fiber in the diet, and an inadequate energy expenditure.

With a basic knowledge of foods and nutrients, Americans can choose a balanced diet that combines the dietary advantages of many cultures. However, for most Americans, achieving a balanced diet is not the only concern. Other related topics, such as the avoidance of obesity, the role of vitamin supplements, and the nutritional value of foods produced by modern methods, are also relevant. Scientists know that dietary requirements vary by age, too. The second section of this chapter, ARE YOU ON THE RIGHT PATH TO A HEALTHY DIET?, will tell you where these issues are addressed in this volume.

WORLD DIETS AND HEALTH

WORKING WITH NATURE

In the early civilizations of the Middle East, India, China, and central America, farmers experimented with the plants that grew there naturally. These plants have been modified by selective breeding to produce bigger yields and to be resistant to disease. In any region the staple food – the main source of carbohydrate and thus of energy – is based on a plant that is natural or adapted to the local environment.

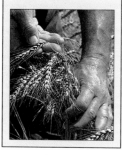

Staple foods
Grains, roots, tubers, and legumes (peas and beans) are utilized as staples in different parts of the world because of their high content of complex carbohydrates (starches), which provide energy. Staples vary in their content of other nutrients, and thus in their overall nutritional value. The sizes of the bags of staples are shown here in proportion to their production worldwide.

The diets people follow today differ from one region of the world to another and also differ from those of our ancestors. Primitive humans survived by hunting and gathering, eating whatever they could find – small animals, birds, or reptiles, and nuts, fruits, berries, or roots. Some tribal communities in Africa, Australia, and South America still live in this way. About 10,000 years ago, humans began to cultivate and harvest crops. Today, most diets around the world are based on a local plant, or staple crop, as the main source of energy.

ENERGY AND PROTEIN SOURCES

For most of the tropics the staple food is rice (or, in parts of Africa, cassava and yams). In much of Europe and North America the staples are wheat, oats, and corn. Other staples include potatoes, yams, peas and beans, peanuts, breadfruit, plantains, and cereal grains such as barley and rye. And in each region there is a cuisine – dishes prepared in a traditional way – that is based on the local staple and on local sources of protein, fats, vegetables, and spices.

Protein sources

Meat, a major source of protein in industrialized countries, is a luxury for much of the world's population, who get their protein from grains, beans and peas, or dairy sources. Many people live on a lacto-ovovegetarian diet, which permits dairy products and eggs but excludes fish and meat. Others rely on fish for their protein. This fish varies from pink salmon to the white flesh of cod, haddock, and turbot eaten in northern latitudes to that of snapper, grouper, and shellfish and the squid and octopus found in warmer waters.

980 MILLION TONS

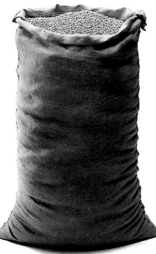

700 MILLION TONS

540 MILLION TONS

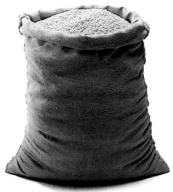

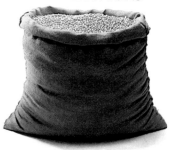

Wheat
More wheat is grown than any other staple. Wheat contains protein, some vitamins and minerals, and carbohydrates, though its nutritional value is reduced by refining.

Rice
Vast quantities of rice are grown in southeast Asia. Although rice has a high energy value, its vitamin and mineral content is reduced when the husk is removed. The same is true of other grains.

Corn
Corn is grown in the Americas, southern Europe, Africa, and east Asia, often in areas where other grains cannot be raised. It is nutritious, though not as rich in protein or minerals as wheat.

TWO DIETS COMPARED

The illustrations below show some of the differences between the American and Japanese diets. The higher prevalence of obesity, adult onset (non-insulin-dependent) diabetes, and coronary heart disease in the US, compared with the prevalence in Japan, is associated with a diet in which fats and sugars contribute a greater proportion of the total calories. Other factors, such as exercise patterns, may also contribute to the differing prevalence of disease.

☐ **Contribution (in kilocalories) of different nutrients to total energy intake**

☐ **Contribution (in kilocalories) of food shown to energy intake**

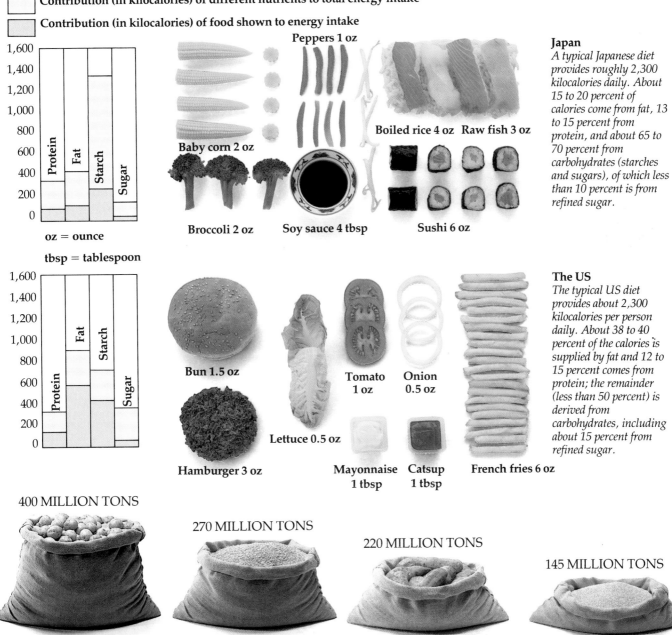

oz = ounce

tbsp = tablespoon

Peppers 1 oz

Baby corn 2 oz

Broccoli 2 oz   **Soy sauce 4 tbsp**

Boiled rice 4 oz   **Raw fish 3 oz**

Sushi 6 oz

Japan
A typical Japanese diet provides roughly 2,300 kilocalories daily. About 15 to 20 percent of calories come from fat, 13 to 15 percent from protein, and about 65 to 70 percent from carbohydrates (starches and sugars), of which less than 10 percent is from refined sugar.

Bun 1.5 oz

Hamburger 3 oz

Lettuce 0.5 oz

Tomato 1 oz   **Onion 0.5 oz**

Mayonnaise 1 tbsp   **Catsup 1 tbsp**   **French fries 6 oz**

The US
The typical US diet provides about 2,300 kilocalories per person daily. About 38 to 40 percent of the calories is supplied by fat and 12 to 15 percent comes from protein; the remainder (less than 50 percent) is derived from carbohydrates, including about 15 percent from refined sugar.

400 MILLION TONS

270 MILLION TONS

220 MILLION TONS

145 MILLION TONS

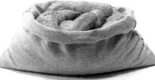

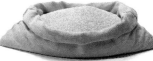

Potatoes
Grown in the cooler latitudes of North America, Europe, and Asia, potatoes contain vitamins and minerals in addition to carbohydrates. Potato skins contain minimal protein.

Barley and rye
Barley is the staple grain in North Africa and parts of Asia. Rye is eaten in central and eastern Europe. Both contain protein, vitamins, minerals, and carbohydrate.

Tropical root crops
Cassava, yams, and sweet potatoes are grown in Africa and South America. They are rich in carbohydrates, vitamins, and minerals, but, like plantain, are low in protein.

Millets
Millets are grown in India, Africa, South America, northern China, and Russia. Millets contain a moderate amount of protein and some vitamins and minerals.

INADEQUATE DIET

Millions of people worldwide do not get enough to eat. Disorders such as kwashiorkor (protein deficiency), as shown below, and marasmus (both calorie and protein deficiency) develop and there is a severe risk of starvation and death. Vitamin deficiencies cause problems ranging from blindness to skin disorders. The combination of poor nutrition and its negative impact on the immune system means that common infectious diseases, such as measles, can kill more easily.

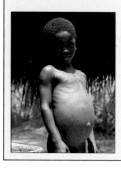

DIET AND DISEASE

How then are these variations in diet reflected in variations in health or disease? First, lack of food is the major contributing factor to poor health in many countries throughout the world. However, when we look at societies in which most of the population have enough to eat, there are still enormous differences in disease patterns from one region to another that may, in part, relate to dietary variations.

Coronary heart disease

There are wide variations in the annual incidence of coronary heart disease. Deaths from coronary heart disease in men 55 to 64 vary from about 800 per 100,000 in parts of northern Europe (such as Scotland) to 280 per 100,000 in Italy and about 60 per 100,000 in Japan. In the US the figure is about 450 per 100,000. For women in the same age range the variation worldwide is from about five per 100,000 to 300 per 100,000.

At first glance, you might think that these variations are due primarily to genetic variations in susceptibility to coronary heart disease – that the risk is determined by genetic factors more common in northern Europeans and Americans than in Italians and Japanese. In fact, genes do play some part. However, some of the differences are considered to be cultural rather than genetic. Statistics show that, when Japanese and Italians come to live in the US and settle into the American way of life, their children (when they become adults) have similar rates of coronary heart disease to the rest of the American population.

Of the various cultural factors that might be responsible for the differences in these rates, researchers have pointed to dietary factors as significant. In countries with high rates of coronary heart disease, there tends to be a high proportion of fat in the diet; in countries with low rates of coronary heart disease, the proportion of fat in the diet tends to be lower. Thus, whereas in Japan rice, fish, and vegetables dominate the diet, and fat represents only one fifth of the calories, in the US meat and dairy products are more often included in the diet and fat accounts for about 38 percent of the total calories consumed – about twice the Japanese level.

It is impossible to be certain that the crucial difference among countries with different rates of coronary heart disease is in the amount of fat in the diet; an association between a high fat intake and a high rate of coronary heart disease does

Goiter
The worldwide occurrence of iodine-deficiency goiter exemplifies the influence of diet on disease. In many mountainous regions, and on certain alluvial plains, such as around the Great Lakes, the soil contains no iodine. If the people of these regions rely solely on locally produced foods, they lack iodine. In areas within developed countries where iodine-deficiency goiter was once prevalent (such as the Midwest), goiter has virtually disappeared.

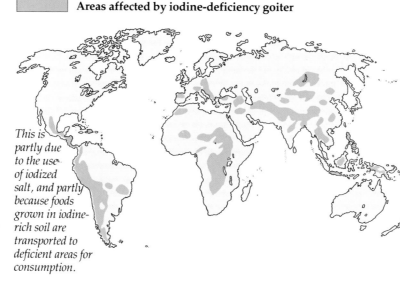

Areas affected by iodine-deficiency goiter

This is partly due to the use of iodized salt, and partly because foods grown in iodine-rich soil are transported to deficient areas for consumption.

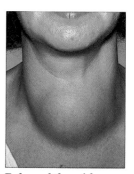

Enlarged thyroid
If a person's iodine intake drops below a certain level, the thyroid gland enlarges (producing a goiter) to maintain its output of iodine-containing thyroid hormones.

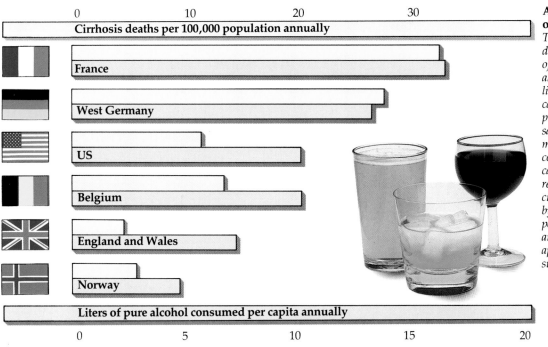

0   10   20   30

Cirrhosis deaths per 100,000 population annually

France

West Germany

US

Belgium

England and Wales

Norway

Liters of pure alcohol consumed per capita annually

0   5   10   15   20

Alcoholic cirrhosis of the liver
The chart compares the death rates (per 100,000 of the population) from alcoholic cirrhosis of the liver and the annual per capita consumption of pure alcohol in several sample countries. The more the people of a country drink, the more cases of cirrhosis are reported. The incidence of cirrhosis is also affected by the number of years a person has drunk heavily and by gender (women appear to be more susceptible than men).

not prove that one causes the other. It could be that other diet-linked factors, such as differences in the total calories consumed, or nondietary factors, such as the amount people exercise, the amount people smoke, or the way different people handle stress, are equally important. Nevertheless, research studies suggest that a reduction in the consumption of fat reduces the risk of coronary heart disease.

Stroke and hypertension

In developed countries such as the US, most people show a gradual rise in blood pressure with age. One of the complications of persistent high blood pressure (hypertension) is stroke. Stroke is a common cause of death in people over 70, although it is becoming less common due to better treatment of hypertension. By contrast, in the rural communities of developing countries, even the very old often have low blood pressure and strokes are rare. Hypertension is virtually unknown in many Pacific islanders, in people who live in the highlands of Papua New Guinea, and in the tribes of the Andes and Amazon.

The explanation for these differences is uncertain, but factors that may be significant include differences in the mineral content of the diets, and the higher level of obesity and stress in people who live in urban populations.

Looking at the mineral factor first, people who live in communities in which blood pressure is found to be low tend to follow a predominantly vegetarian diet that contains little sodium in the form of salt. Some studies have shown that a low ratio of sodium to potassium in the diet may be of benefit. Other studies suggest that increased calcium and magnesium levels are beneficial in preventing mild hypertension. However, some research has shown no relationship and the issue remains obscure. Alcohol, even in relatively small amounts, may be an important factor in hypertension for a susceptible person.

Immigration and health
Studies show that second-generation immigrants have a disease pattern similar to that of the indigenous population. This suggests that life-style (including diet) and environment may play a more significant role than genetic factors in disease patterns around the world.

13

Being overweight is recognized as an important factor for many people who have hypertension. It is clear that one of the benefits of weight loss in people who are seriously overweight is the normalization of blood pressure.

Cancer

Cancer affects people all over the world, but the cancers that are common in some developing countries are often rare in developed or other developing countries and vice versa. Much research being done today is concerned with identifying foods, additives, preservatives, and contaminants that may cause disease. In addition, researchers are studying those nutrients (including vitamin A and its precursors such as carotene) that may decrease the risk of cancer development.

TRADITIONAL AND CONTEMPORARY CUISINE

The variations in the food eaten throughout the world are not the only causative factors in the variation in the patterns of disease from country to country. In this century every developed country has seen substantial changes in the way food is grown, prepared, and stored.

Until recently, the main problem of people living in high latitudes was how to maintain, over the winter, the food harvested during the previous summer and fall. Salting, drying, smoking, and curing of fish and meat became highly developed, while vegetables were salted and made into dishes such as sauerkraut that could be kept for months or years.

Today's foods

These traditional ways of preserving food were in part abandoned with the introduction of refrigeration. In the US and western Europe, where refrigerators and freezers have been in widespread use for more than 50 years, salted and dried foods are used less and smoked foods such as bacon and ham are more lightly preserved than they once were. Furthermore, it appears that people are eating more fresh food. Because fresh foods have a higher vitamin content (since the vitamins have not been lost or destroyed during processing and storage), this factor has improved the quality of our diet. Whether these changes have influenced disease patterns is uncertain and unproven, but in these same countries there has been at least a coincidental steady increase in life expectancy.

Preserved foods
One change in the American diet over the last 50 years has been a reduction in the consumption of smoked, salted, or pickled foods (below). The effects of this possibly beneficial change on health are not proven.

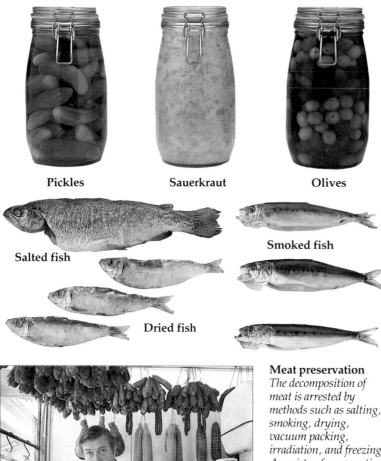

Pickles   Sauerkraut   Olives

Salted fish

Smoked fish

Dried fish

Meat preservation
The decomposition of meat is arrested by methods such as salting, smoking, drying, vacuum packing, irradiation, and freezing. A variety of preservatives are used in making sausages (left). Most hot dogs contain sodium nitrite or nitrate. The safety of these chemicals has been questioned, since they may be converted by stomach acids into cancer-causing nitrosamines.

WHERE DOES OUR FOOD COME FROM?

Americans have an unrivaled availability of high-quality foods. In parts of the US it is possible to buy fruit, vegetables, meat, dairy products, and poultry directly from local farms. In addition, supermarkets offer a bewildering variety of foods, thanks to refrigeration. The introduction of refrigerators into American homes revolutionized the shopping patterns and diets of most Americans, making it possible to enjoy not only specialized items from other states but also exotic foods transported by refrigerated freighters and cargo planes from all over the world. Today, fresh fruits and vegetables are available throughout the year.

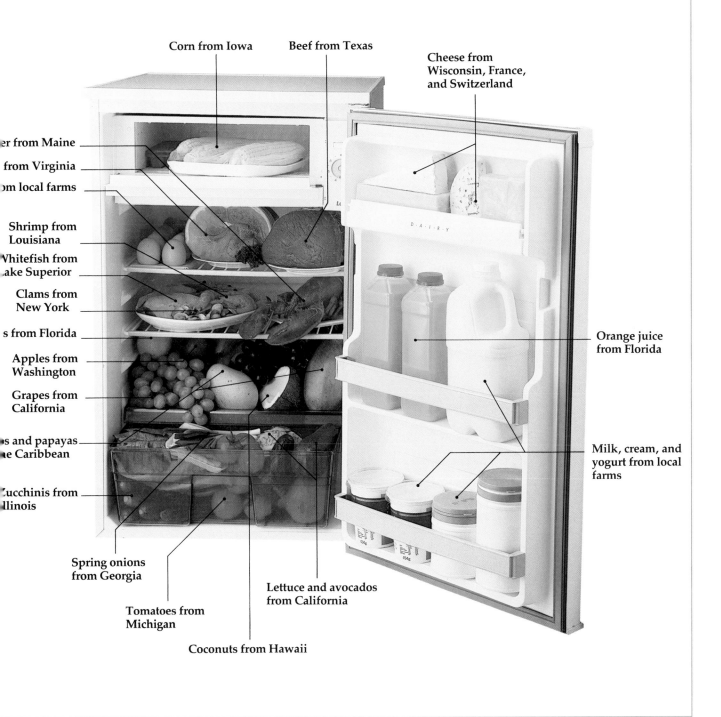

Corn from Iowa

Beef from Texas

Cheese from Wisconsin, France, and Switzerland

er from Maine

from Virginia

om local farms

Shrimp from Louisiana

Whitefish from Lake Superior

Clams from New York

s from Florida

Apples from Washington

Grapes from California

s and papayas e Caribbean

Zucchinis from Illinois

Orange juice from Florida

Milk, cream, and yogurt from local farms

Spring onions from Georgia

Lettuce and avocados from California

Tomatoes from Michigan

Coconuts from Hawaii

ARE YOU ON THE RIGHT PATH TO A HEALTHY DIET?

The first section of this chapter, WORLD DIETS AND HEALTH, raised the question that variations in patterns of disease around the world may be influenced by differences in diet. If these theories are correct, it follows that people who have access to a wide variety of foods can influence their health through greater control of their intake.

Begin by reviewing the primary dietary concerns of people living in the US today. Listed here are six areas for your consideration. Each will direct you to the place in this volume where the issues are addressed more fully.

How good is the quality of your diet?

Nutrition experts agree that the healthiest dietary patterns are those in which people eat the widest possible selection of naturally occurring unrefined foods. There are no bad foods – only bad diets.

A high-quality, balanced diet has two components. First, the diet must be complete, which is to say it must contain sufficient quantities of all the known essential nutrients. Second, the diet should not contain too much of any single dietary component – particularly fat, sugar, or salt – or too many calories overall. Much of Chapter Three, YOU AND YOUR DIET, reviews ways in which you can improve the quality of your diet. The section on BALANCING YOUR DIET offers methods to ensure you get all the right nutrients, while AVOIDING EXCESS points out the risks of overeating.

Nutritional information
Finding a good "map" of optimum nutrition is the first step in successfully reorienting your diet.

DECLINE AND DECAY

HEALTH AND VITALITY

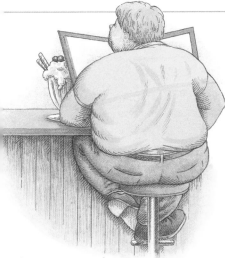

Are you eating too much?

Surveys performed by the National Center for Health Statistics indicate that one in every ten Americans (i.e., more than 20 million people) is more than 20 percent heavier than his or her optimum weight. These figures underscore the fact that, for a substantial number of people in the US and many other developed countries, the primary diet-related problem is not a deficiency of nutrients. It is simply the problem of eating far too much and expending too few calories.

Obesity increases the risk of health problems such as hyper-tension (high blood pressure), diabetes mellitus, high blood cholesterol, and coronary artery and gallbladder disease.

How do people become over-weight? Because they ingest more calories than they expend in physical activity. The reasons *why* they eat too much in relation to their activity levels, and what they can do about it, are more complex. The question of over-eating, the causes and medical effects of obesity, and methods of weight control are covered in Chapter Four, DIET AND YOUR WEIGHT.

Should you supplement your diet?

Surveys by the Food and Drug Administration show that about half the population take vitamin and/or mineral supplements.

If your diet is balanced, supplements are not required. In the distant past, children of even the relatively affluent were at risk of vitamin deficiencies, especially in the winter. However, overall, today's fresh food supply has eliminated the deficiency disorders of old. These included scurvy, rickets, and beriberi, caused by a lack of vitamins; goiter, from lack of iodine; and impaired growth, due to lack of calories and protein.

There are, however, still large numbers of poorer people with marginal food intakes and dietary deficiency. Many children and adult women are deficient in iron. Vitamin B_1 (thiamine) and vitamin C deficiencies are not uncommon among alcoholics and some elderly persons.

The sections on VITAMINS AND MINERALS in Chapter Two, BALANCING YOUR DIET in Chapter Three, and VITAMIN AND MINERAL DEFICIENCIES and OSTEOPOROSIS in Chapter Five will help you decide whether you need to take a supplement.

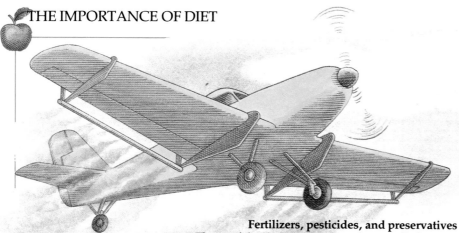

Fertilizers, pesticides, and preservatives
The use of chemicals in agriculture dramatically increases yields, resulting in cheaper foods for the consumer. Preservatives prevent spoiling of food by bacteria and molds. Any risk from ingesting chemicals in food must be weighed against the fact that moldy, spoiled food is also a health hazard.

Is food produced by modern methods safe?

Food today is plentiful and varied, but little of it comes to the table in its "natural" form. The cereals, fruits, and vegetables we eat are treated with pesticides and packaged using preservatives, colorings, and flavor enhancers. The chickens, turkeys, and cattle that provide much of our animal protein are often raised with the aid of hormones and growth enhancers.

Concerns about the safety of food produced today fall into two areas. First, many people are concerned about the substances added to food – believing, for example, that they may cause cancers, allergies, or hyperactivity in children.

Irradiated food
Irradiation does not make food radioactive. However, the food's structure is altered slightly. Bacterial growth is arrested and preservation is enhanced.

In reaction to these claims, a vociferous, growing minority of people have campaigned for the production of natural "organic" food that has been grown without pesticides and is free of chemical preservatives, colorings, and hormones.

A second area of concern is the apparent increase in food poisoning in the US and elsewhere from bacterial contamina-

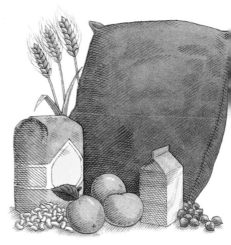

tion of food. This results not from the availability of modern food technology, but from its faulty application. One solution offered to reduce cases of food poisoning and facilitate preservation – the irradiation of food – is itself an area of controversy.

The sections on FOOD TECHNOLOGY in Chapter Two, on FOOD STORAGE AND PREPARATION in Chapter Three, on DIET AND CANCER, FOOD ALLERGY AND FOOD INTOLERANCE, and FOOD POISONING in Chapter Five address many of these concerns. On the whole,

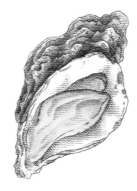

scientists working in the field of food safety and hygiene remain convinced that the food industry is doing a good job. Chilled, preserved, canned, and frozen foods that are properly prepared and marketed within their "sell by" dates are safer by far than natural foods that may have been stored in unmonitored storage facilities. Modern processing methods also allow a variety of foods to be more affordable than their fresh counterparts. For some people, the ideal would be

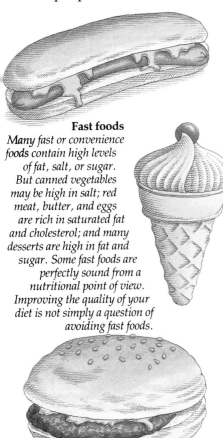

Fast foods
Many fast or convenience foods contain high levels of fat, salt, or sugar. But canned vegetables may be high in salt; red meat, butter, and eggs are rich in saturated fat and cholesterol; and many desserts are high in fat and sugar. Some fast foods are perfectly sound from a nutritional point of view. Improving the quality of your diet is not simply a question of avoiding fast foods.

to raise chickens and vegetables themselves. However, for most of us, this is unrealistic. Mass production and mass marketing have supplied a growing population with safe, wholesome, and less expensive foods, in and out of season.

Is your eating behavior healthy?

Over the past 30 to 40 years, eating habits have changed. Some see the change resulting largely from increased pressures – from work commitments and leisure activities – on our use of time. Whereas at one time a day's food was traditionally eaten in "three square meals," with the family, now some people eat a running succession of smaller meals. Others eat little or nothing during the day and then consume a full day's calories in the evening.

Some families never sit down together at a table to eat a traditional meal. Some people have dispensed with using a table altogether, instead eating much of their food at less traditional places such as the office desk or the park bench or in front of the TV. This is a reflection of our changing social eating patterns.

The section on EATING BEHAVIOR in Chapter Three examines the effects on health of how we eat. The overall message is that eating a succession of numerous small meals is not a danger to health. In fact, it may be beneficial. The nutritional content is of greatest importance. Many convenience and fast foods have a high content of fat, sugar, and salt, and are also low in fiber and certain vitamins. However, if much of your diet consists of snack or convenience foods, there are ways of ensuring dietary quality.

Social eating
Meals eaten at a table with family or friends provide an important social quality to the biological process of eating.

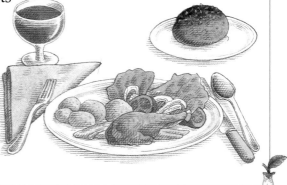

The oyster myth
There is no evidence that eating oysters leads to sexual arousal or has any effect on sexual potency.

Should you believe everything you read and hear about diet and nutrition?

Advice on nutrition and diet is a huge industry in the US today, and the marketing and selling of new products that are "high" or "low" in various nutrients is big business. However, many advertisements are designed to sell products rather than to provide helpful information about nutrition. Much of the advice is conflicting, confusing, or inaccurate. It may be based on inconclusive research that is used to promote the product at the expense of the public's desire to live and eat in as healthy a way as possible.

The section in Chapter Three on MYTH AND REALITY is designed to help you sort out some of the facts from the fallacies on nutritional matters.

CHAPTER TWO

FOOD AND NUTRIENTS

IF YOU ARE LIKE MANY Americans, you are more conscious than ever about the foods you and your family eat. However, it can be difficult to translate dietary advice – such as getting enough calcium for your bones or reducing the fat in your diet – into the food you eat. Any attempt to rectify a dietary imbalance can create another imbalance unless you understand the basic nutrients your body needs to function and the types of foods that can provide you with these nutrients.

The opening section of this chapter, WHAT IS FOOD?, is a pictorial introduction to the primary food groups and the nutrients they contain. The processes by which the body uses nutrients, called metabolism, are complex. Metabolism has two primary aspects, catabolism and anabolism. Catabolism consists of the processes that break down complex body chemicals into simpler substances or that release energy for the functioning of body cells. Anabolism consists of all the processes that build up structural components for energy storage and for the body's growth and repair. The section in this chapter on FOOD FOR ENERGY AND GROWTH describes how the carbohydrates, fats, and proteins in the food you eat provide the bulk

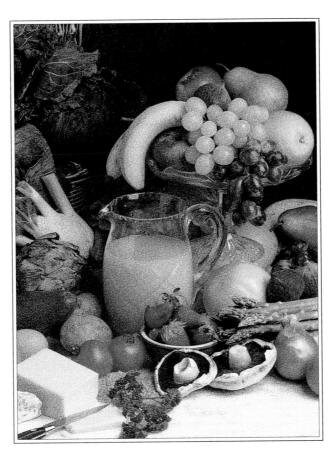

of the fuel for catabolism and the building blocks for anabolic processes.

As explained in the section on VITAMINS AND MINERALS, small amounts of 13 vitamins are required for growth and repair mechanisms. In addition, 16 different minerals have an essential role as facilitators of metabolism; some of them (such as calcium and phosphorus) also provide the raw materials for processes such as bone formation. When we are healthy, our bodies are highly efficient at conserving and recycling these essential substances. The vitamins and minerals that we ingest are used to replace the normal losses that occur in excretion, sweat, and blood loss.

Two other essential components of our dietary intake are fiber and water. Fiber – found in all fruits and vegetables – aids the work of the digestive system. Water replaces the fluids that are continually being lost from the body in sweat and urine. These valuable substances are reviewed in the section on FIBER AND WATER. The section on THE DIGESTIVE PROCESS reviews in detail how nutrients are released from food in the alimentary tract, broken down, and absorbed into the bloodstream. Finally, FOOD TECHNOLOGY examines some production and processing methods.

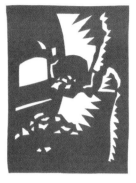

WHAT IS FOOD?

FOOD HAS MANY FACES – it provides a pleasurable stimulus to the palate, has a role in many social and religious rituals, and adds color to the home and marketplace. In a limited chemical sense, food can be defined as any solid or liquid that provides the body with energy and with materials for growth, repair, and reproduction. The substances in food that fulfill these functions are called nutrients.

There are two main types of nutrients – macronutrients (carbohydrates, fats, and proteins) and micronutrients (vitamins and minerals). Hardly any foods contain only one nutrient. Most unprocessed foods are complex mixtures, composed mainly of macronutrients in varying proportions, with tiny amounts of micronutrients.

Food also contains water and fiber, two vital substances that are sometimes considered macronutrients because the amount of them contained in foods is large relative to vitamins and minerals. These components are discussed in FIBER AND WATER on page 48.

FOOD DIGESTION

Food is broken down (digested) in the stomach and intestines. The nutrients are then absorbed into the bloodstream. In general, macronutrients consist of large molecules that must be broken down into smaller molecules before they can be absorbed. Water and most micronutrients can be absorbed directly. Fiber is composed of substances, largely complex carbohydrates, that escape digestion in the small intestine (although some fiber is fermented by bacteria in the large intestine). Fiber influences the digestion, absorption, and metabolism of many nutrients.

Esophagus
Stomach
Small intestine
Large intestine

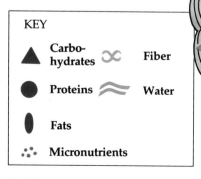

1 The mechanical breakdown of food, along with some digestion of starch, begins in the mouth.

2 In the stomach, more mechanical breakdown occurs and the digestion of protein and fat begins.

3 The main processes of digestion, and the absorption of all nutrients and water, take place in the small intestine.

4 Some water and salts are absorbed into the bloodstream from the large intestine.

5 Fiber passes through the small intestine and, either unaltered or partially fermented, forms part of the bulk of feces.

KEY

▲ Carbohydrates
∞ Fiber
● Proteins
≈ Water
◗ Fats
∴ Micronutrients

THE ESSENTIAL NUTRIENTS

MACRONUTRIENTS

Macronutrients are substances needed in substantial quantities by the body. Macronutrients, and the foods that provide them, are discussed further in FOOD FOR ENERGY AND GROWTH on page 30.

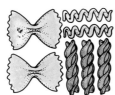

Carbohydrates, which include starches and sugars, are the primary energy sources.

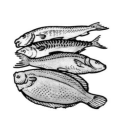

Fats provide energy in a more concentrated form than carbohydrates. They also supply the essential fatty acids needed for growth, tissue repair, and the creation of chemical messengers (prostaglandins).

Proteins primarily provide materials (amino acids) for body growth and repair. Under certain conditions, proteins supply energy.

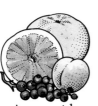

MICRONUTRIENTS

Micronutrients are substances needed in relatively small (or very small) quantities by the body. Micronutrients, and the foods that provide them, are discussed further in VITAMINS AND MINERALS on page 36.

Vitamins facilitate a variety of processes, including the production of energy inside body cells and the growth and division of cells. A total of 13 vitamins must be provided by the diet (some can be made in the body, but usually not in sufficient quantities).

Minerals are chemical elements, such as calcium and iron, required by the body for growth or to facilitate essential body processes. There are 16 minerals that must be provided by the diet.

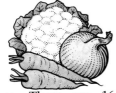

THE COMPONENTS OF A SAMPLE FOOD

There is no "typical" food, but an ear of corn offers an idea of the relative amounts of macronutrients, micronutrients, water, fiber, and other substances contained in a food. Water and macronutrients form the largest part of most foods; micronutrients are present in very small quantities. Fiber is found to varying degrees, but only in foods of plant origin.

**Water
74 percent**

**Macronutrients
(carbohydrates, fats, and proteins)
20 percent**

**Dietary fiber
5 percent**

**Other substances
1 percent or less**

**Micronutrients
(vitamins and minerals)
0.1 percent or less**

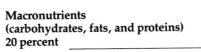

NUTRIENT CONTENT OF SOME COMMON FOODS

The following six pages show some common foods from a variety of food groups. The energy content (in kilocalories) and the amounts of protein, carbohydrate, fat, and dietary fiber for a typical serving size are given, as are the vitamins and minerals that are present in significant amounts. For foods in which the fat content is significant, a breakdown into saturated, monounsaturated, and polyunsaturated fats is listed. Otherwise, the total fat content is given.

UNITS OF FOOD ENERGY

The standard unit of food energy is the calorie. However, 1 calorie represents an extremely small amount of energy. The "calorie" that most people "count" refers to a kilocalorie (1,000 calories), which is also sometimes written as a Calorie (with a capital C). Food energy values throughout this book are given in kilocalories (kcal), but remember that a kilocalorie is exactly the same as the Calorie of popular usage.

MEAT AND POULTRY

Meat and poultry are important sources of protein, minerals, and B vitamins. A disadvantage is that even lean meats contain saturated fat. In general, skinless poultry contains less fat (including saturated fat) than lean meat; at the same time, it provides an important source of protein. Removing the skin always reduces the fat content. Remember, however, that poultry contains far less iron – an important part of the diet for menstruating women – than red meat.

ORGAN MEAT LIVER
Similar examples:
brain, heart, kidney, sweetbread

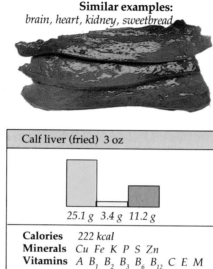

KEY			
☐ Protein		☐ Monounsaturated	
☐ Carbohydrate		fat	
☐ Total fat		☐ Polyunsaturated fat	
☐ Saturated fat		☐ Dietary fiber	

KEY TO VITAMINS

B_1	thiamine	B_6	pyridoxine
B_2	riboflavin	B_{12}	cyanocobalamin
B_3	niacin	M	folic acid

KEY TO MINERALS

Ca	calcium	Mg	magnesium
Cu	copper	Na	sodium
F	fluorine	P	phosphorus
Fe	iron	S	sulfur
I	iodine	Se	selenium
K	potassium	Zn	zinc

KEY TO WEIGHTS AND MEASURES

$kcal$	kilocalorie	$tbsp$	tablespoon
g	gram	oz	ounce

Calf liver (fried) 3 oz

25.1 g   3.4 g   11.2 g

Calories	222 kcal
Minerals	Cu Fe K P S Zn
Vitamins	A B_1 B_2 B_3 B_6 B_{12} C E M

LEAN MEAT BEEF
Similar examples:
lamb, pork, veal

POULTRY CHICKEN
Similar examples: *duck, goose, turkey*

EGGS

Eggs are an excellent source of protein and of several vitamins and minerals. Eggs also contain cholesterol. However, the contribution of dietary cholesterol to the overall concentration of cholesterol in your blood is minor compared to that made by saturated fats. Eggs also contain saturated fat – and should be limited to no more than four per week.

EGGS

**Sirloin steak
(broiled, trimmed of fat) 3 oz**

27.4 g   3.1 g   2.9 g   0.1 g

Calories	176 kcal
Minerals	Fe K P S Zn
Vitamins	B_1 B_3 B_6 B_{12} K

**Chicken
(roasted, skinless white meat) 3 oz**

26.9 g   0.9 g   1.1 g   0.6 g

Calories	141 kcal
Minerals	K P S Zn
Vitamins	B_2 B_3

Egg 1 large raw

6.5 g   0.5 g   1.8 g   2.5 g   0.4 g

Calories	82 kcal
Minerals	Fe P S Zn
Vitamins	A B_2 B_{12} D E

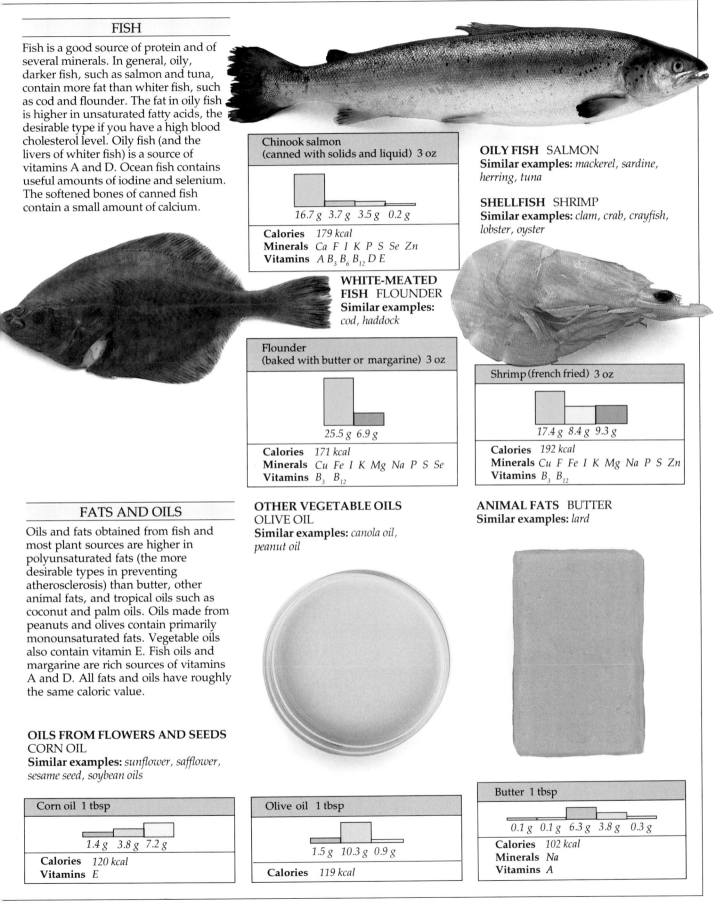

FISH

Fish is a good source of protein and of several minerals. In general, oily, darker fish, such as salmon and tuna, contain more fat than whiter fish, such as cod and flounder. The fat in oily fish is higher in unsaturated fatty acids, the desirable type if you have a high blood cholesterol level. Oily fish (and the livers of whiter fish) is a source of vitamins A and D. Ocean fish contains useful amounts of iodine and selenium. The softened bones of canned fish contain a small amount of calcium.

Chinook salmon (canned with solids and liquid) 3 oz

16.7 g   3.7 g   3.5 g   0.2 g

Calories	179 kcal
Minerals	Ca F I K P S Se Zn
Vitamins	A B_3 B_6 B_{12} D E

OILY FISH SALMON
Similar examples: *mackerel, sardine, herring, tuna*

SHELLFISH SHRIMP
Similar examples: *clam, crab, crayfish, lobster, oyster*

WHITE-MEATED FISH FLOUNDER
Similar examples: *cod, haddock*

Flounder (baked with butter or margarine) 3 oz

25.5 g   6.9 g

Calories	171 kcal
Minerals	Cu Fe I K Mg Na P S Se
Vitamins	B_3 B_{12}

Shrimp (french fried) 3 oz

17.4 g   8.4 g   9.3 g

Calories	192 kcal
Minerals	Cu F Fe I K Mg Na P S Zn
Vitamins	B_3 B_{12}

FATS AND OILS

Oils and fats obtained from fish and most plant sources are higher in polyunsaturated fats (the more desirable types in preventing atherosclerosis) than butter, other animal fats, and tropical oils such as coconut and palm oils. Oils made from peanuts and olives contain primarily monounsaturated fats. Vegetable oils also contain vitamin E. Fish oils and margarine are rich sources of vitamins A and D. All fats and oils have roughly the same caloric value.

OTHER VEGETABLE OILS
OLIVE OIL
Similar examples: *canola oil, peanut oil*

ANIMAL FATS BUTTER
Similar examples: *lard*

OILS FROM FLOWERS AND SEEDS
CORN OIL
Similar examples: *sunflower, safflower, sesame seed, soybean oils*

Corn oil 1 tbsp

1.4 g   3.8 g   7.2 g

Calories	120 kcal
Vitamins	E

Olive oil 1 tbsp

1.5 g   10.3 g   0.9 g

Calories	119 kcal

Butter 1 tbsp

0.1 g   0.1 g   6.3 g   3.8 g   0.3 g

Calories	102 kcal
Minerals	Na
Vitamins	A

25

DAIRY PRODUCTS

Cow's milk is the single most complete food. It contains most of the essential nutrients, though it is a relatively poor source of vitamin C and iron. Skim milk and 2% milk contain less fat than whole milk. Hard cheeses such as cheddar are a good source of protein and calcium, as well as vitamin A and riboflavin. They also have a large amount of sodium, saturated fat, and cholesterol and are a concentrated source of energy (calories).

WHOLE MILK

SKIM MILK

YOGURT

HARD CHEESE

2% MILK

HALF AND HALF

COTTAGE CHEESE

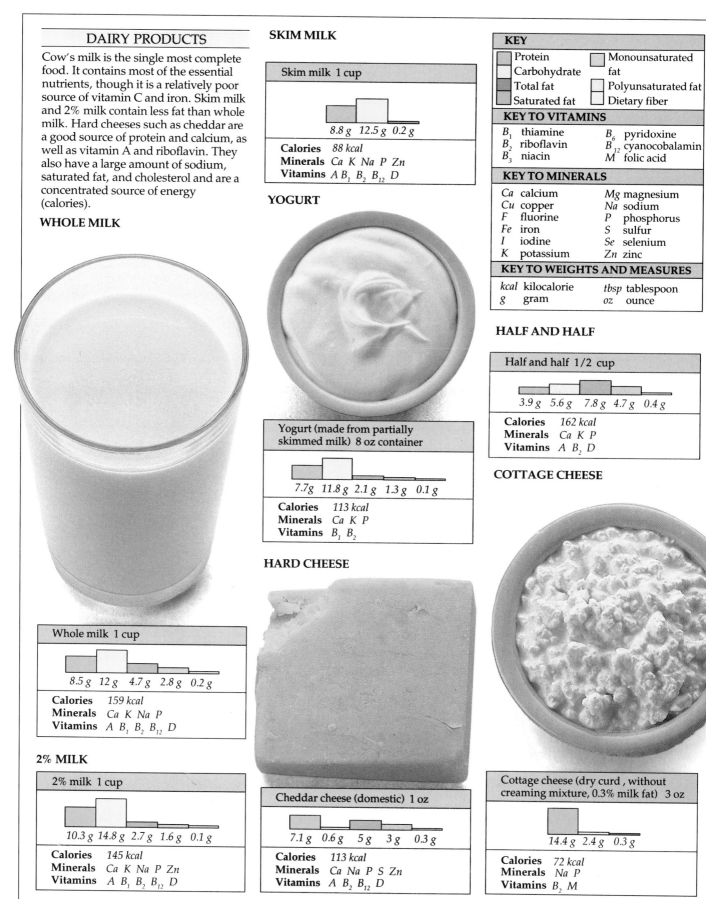

KEY

Protein	Monounsaturated fat
Carbohydrate	
Total fat	Polyunsaturated fat
Saturated fat	Dietary fiber

KEY TO VITAMINS

B_1	thiamine	B_6	pyridoxine
B_2	riboflavin	B_{12}	cyanocobalamin
B_3	niacin	M	folic acid

KEY TO MINERALS

Ca	calcium	Mg	magnesium
Cu	copper	Na	sodium
F	fluorine	P	phosphorus
Fe	iron	S	sulfur
I	iodine	Se	selenium
K	potassium	Zn	zinc

KEY TO WEIGHTS AND MEASURES

| $kcal$ | kilocalorie | $tbsp$ | tablespoon |
| g | gram | oz | ounce |

Skim milk 1 cup

8.8 g   12.5 g   0.2 g

Calories	88 kcal
Minerals	Ca K Na P Zn
Vitamins	A B_1 B_2 B_{12} D

Yogurt (made from partially skimmed milk) 8 oz container

7.7 g   11.8 g   2.1 g   1.3 g   0.1 g

Calories	113 kcal
Minerals	Ca K P
Vitamins	B_1 B_2

Whole milk 1 cup

8.5 g   12 g   4.7 g   2.8 g   0.2 g

Calories	159 kcal
Minerals	Ca K Na P
Vitamins	A B_1 B_2 B_{12} D

2% milk 1 cup

10.3 g   14.8 g   2.7 g   1.6 g   0.1 g

Calories	145 kcal
Minerals	Ca K Na P Zn
Vitamins	A B_1 B_2 B_{12} D

Cheddar cheese (domestic) 1 oz

7.1 g   0.6 g   5 g   3 g   0.3 g

Calories	113 kcal
Minerals	Ca Na P S Zn
Vitamins	A B_2 B_{12} D

Half and half 1/2 cup

3.9 g   5.6 g   7.8 g   4.7 g   0.4 g

Calories	162 kcal
Minerals	Ca K P
Vitamins	A B_2 D

Cottage cheese (dry curd, without creaming mixture, 0.3% milk fat) 3 oz

14.4 g   2.4 g   0.3 g

Calories	72 kcal
Minerals	Na P
Vitamins	B_2 M

FRUITS

Many fruits, such as oranges, grapefruits, cantaloupes, and strawberries, are excellent sources of vitamin C. Some fruits, such as oranges, apricots, and peaches, provide vitamin A. Fruits also contain fiber and some energy in the form of the sugars fructose and sucrose. Dried fruits provide more concentrated amounts of energy and vitamin A, but relatively little vitamin C. Some dried fruits such as apricots, figs, dates, raisins, and prunes contain iron and potassium.

BERRIES STRAWBERRY
Similar examples:
blueberry, cranberry, raspberry

FRUITS WITH PITS PEACH
Similar examples: *apricot, cherry*

Peach (1 medium, 2.5 inches in diameter)			
0.6 g	9.7 g	0.1 g	1 g
Calories	38 kcal		
Minerals	K		
Vitamins	A C		

WINE

Table wine (12.2% alcohol by volume, 9.9% by weight) 3.5 fluid oz glass	
0.1 g	4.3 g
Calories	87 kcal
Minerals	Fe

CITRUS FRUITS ORANGE
Similar examples: *grapefruit, lemon, lime*

Florida orange (1 medium, 2.7 inches in diameter)			
1.1 g	18.1 g	0.3 g	4 g
Calories	71 kcal		
Minerals	K		
Vitamins	A B₁ C M		

SUGAR

Sugar (beet or cane, granulated) 1 tbsp
11.9 g
Calories   46 kcal

Strawberries (fresh) 1 cup			
1 g	12.5 g	0.7 g	3 g
Calories	55 kcal		
Minerals	Fe K		
Vitamins	C		

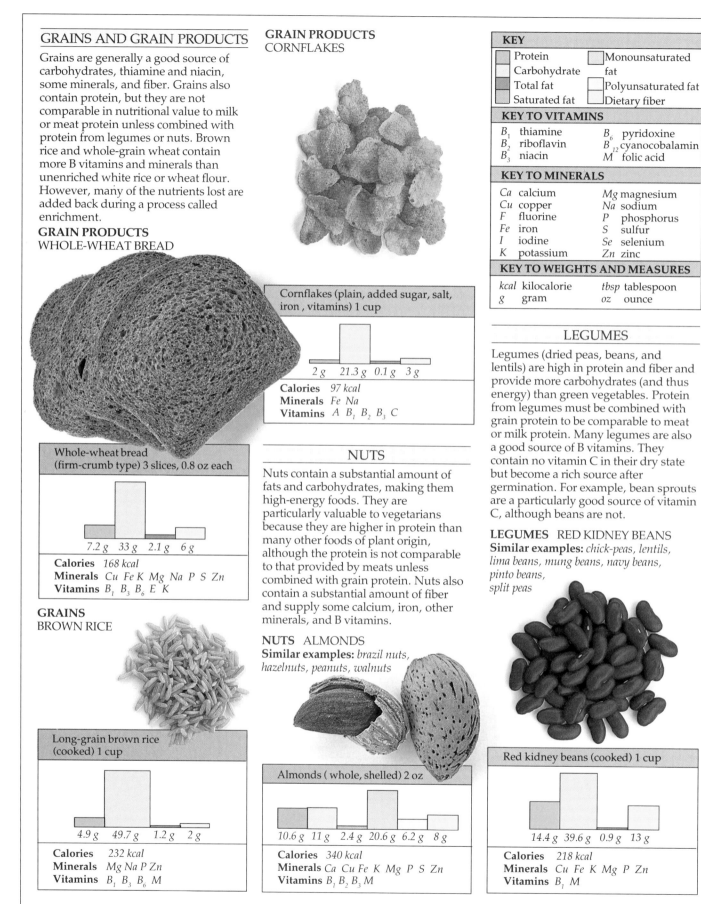

GRAINS AND GRAIN PRODUCTS

Grains are generally a good source of carbohydrates, thiamine and niacin, some minerals, and fiber. Grains also contain protein, but they are not comparable in nutritional value to milk or meat protein unless combined with protein from legumes or nuts. Brown rice and whole-grain wheat contain more B vitamins and minerals than unenriched white rice or wheat flour. However, many of the nutrients lost are added back during a process called enrichment.

GRAIN PRODUCTS
WHOLE-WHEAT BREAD

Whole-wheat bread
(firm-crumb type) 3 slices, 0.8 oz each

| 7.2 g | 33 g | 2.1 g | 6 g |

Calories 168 kcal
Minerals Cu Fe K Mg Na P S Zn
Vitamins B_1 B_3 B_6 E K

GRAINS
BROWN RICE

Long-grain brown rice
(cooked) 1 cup

| 4.9 g | 49.7 g | 1.2 g | 2 g |

Calories 232 kcal
Minerals Mg Na P Zn
Vitamins B_1 B_3 B_6 M

GRAIN PRODUCTS
CORNFLAKES

Cornflakes (plain, added sugar, salt, iron , vitamins) 1 cup

| 2 g | 21.3 g | 0.1 g | 3 g |

Calories 97 kcal
Minerals Fe Na
Vitamins A B_1 B_2 B_3 C

NUTS

Nuts contain a substantial amount of fats and carbohydrates, making them high-energy foods. They are particularly valuable to vegetarians because they are higher in protein than many other foods of plant origin, although the protein is not comparable to that provided by meats unless combined with grain protein. Nuts also contain a substantial amount of fiber and supply some calcium, iron, other minerals, and B vitamins.

NUTS ALMONDS
Similar examples: *brazil nuts, hazelnuts, peanuts, walnuts*

Almonds (whole, shelled) 2 oz

| 10.6 g | 11 g | 2.4 g | 20.6 g | 6.2 g | 8 g |

Calories 340 kcal
Minerals Ca Cu Fe K Mg P S Zn
Vitamins B_1 B_2 B_3 M

KEY

Protein		Monounsaturated fat
Carbohydrate		
Total fat		Polyunsaturated fat
Saturated fat		Dietary fiber

KEY TO VITAMINS

B_1	thiamine	B_6	pyridoxine
B_2	riboflavin	B_{12}	cyanocobalamin
B_3	niacin	M	folic acid

KEY TO MINERALS

Ca	calcium	Mg	magnesium
Cu	copper	Na	sodium
F	fluorine	P	phosphorus
Fe	iron	S	sulfur
I	iodine	Se	selenium
K	potassium	Zn	zinc

KEY TO WEIGHTS AND MEASURES

kcal	kilocalorie	tbsp	tablespoon
g	gram	oz	ounce

LEGUMES

Legumes (dried peas, beans, and lentils) are high in protein and fiber and provide more carbohydrates (and thus energy) than green vegetables. Protein from legumes must be combined with grain protein to be comparable to meat or milk protein. Many legumes are also a good source of B vitamins. They contain no vitamin C in their dry state but become a rich source after germination. For example, bean sprouts are a particularly good source of vitamin C, although beans are not.

LEGUMES RED KIDNEY BEANS
Similar examples: *chick-peas, lentils, lima beans, mung beans, navy beans, pinto beans, split peas*

Red kidney beans (cooked) 1 cup

| 14.4 g | 39.6 g | 0.9 g | 13 g |

Calories 218 kcal
Minerals Cu Fe K Mg P Zn
Vitamins B_1 M

VEGETABLES

Potatoes and root vegetables such as turnips provide both energy and protein. Vegetable protein cannot substitute for meat or milk protein or even legume-grain or nut-grain protein combinations. Leaf vegetables are a rich source of minerals, vitamins, water, and fiber. Most vegetables are especially valuable when eaten raw, or cooked minimally, so that micronutrients are not lost. Green vegetables provide vitamins A, C, and K and folic acid; carrots, dark green, leafy vegetables and some squashes provide vitamin A. Other root vegetables and potatoes are good sources of vitamin C. Many vegetables contain potassium.

TUBERS POTATO

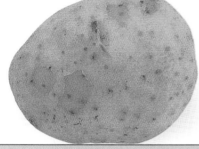

Potato (1 large, baked in skin) 8 oz			
4.6 g	36.9 g	0.15 g	2 g
Calories	163 kcal		
Minerals	Fe K Mg P		
Vitamins	B₁ B₃ B₆ C K		

SEED VEGETABLES TOMATO
Similar examples: *pepper*

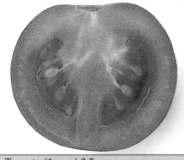

Tomato (1 raw) 3.5 oz			
1 g	4.3 g	0.2 g	1.5 g
Calories	20 kcal		
Minerals	K		
Vitamins	A C K		

SQUASHES
ZUCCHINI
Similar examples:
*acorn squash,
butternut squash,
cucumber, pumpkin*

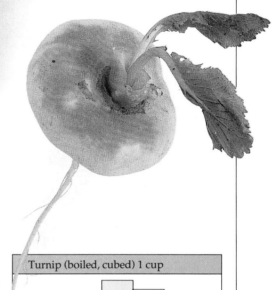

Zucchini (boiled, cubed) 1 cup			
2.1 g	5.3 g	0.2 g	4 g
Calories	25 kcal		
Minerals	K		
Vitamins	A B₁ B₂ B₃ C		

GREEN LEAFY VEGETABLES
SPINACH
Similar examples: *brussels sprouts, greens, broccoli*

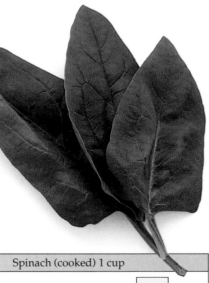

Spinach (cooked) 1 cup			
5.4 g	6.5 g	0.5 g	11 g
Calories	41 kcal		
Minerals	Ca Cu Fe K Mg		
Vitamins	A B₁ B₂ C E K M		

ROOT VEGETABLES TURNIP
Similar examples: *beet, parsnip, radish*

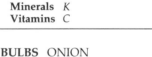

Turnip (boiled, cubed) 1 cup		
1.2 g	7.6 g	3 g
Calories	36 kcal	
Minerals	K	
Vitamins	C	

BULBS ONION
Similar examples: *garlic, leek, scallion, shallot*

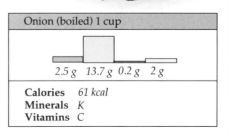

Onion (boiled) 1 cup			
2.5 g	13.7 g	0.2 g	2 g
Calories	61 kcal		
Minerals	K		
Vitamins	C		

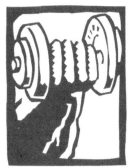

FOOD FOR ENERGY AND GROWTH

GOOD HEALTH is facilitated by obtaining the nutrients that provide your body with energy and with materials for growth, functional activities, repair, and reproduction. The best way to ensure that you receive adequate amounts of all nutrients is to choose from the widest possible selection of naturally occurring foods.

Your body uses carbohydrates and fats as its primary energy sources. Carbohydrates and fats, in addition to proteins, also supply the nutrients that your body needs for growth, functional activities, and maintenance.

CARBOHYDRATES

Carbohydrates are compounds of the elements carbon, hydrogen, and oxygen; they have structures based on simple chemical units called saccharides. These chemical units can be linked together in different ways and in different numbers to form the various types of carbohydrates.

The carbohydrates in food fall into three groups – sugars, starches, and a group that consists of cellulose and related materials. Of these, sugars and starches are used by the body for energy. Cellulose cannot be digested by humans, but only by ruminants such as cows. It forms a major part of dietary fiber.

Sugars in food taste sweet and consist of either single saccharide units (monosaccharides) or two linked units (disaccharides). Starches and cellulose have large molecules consisting of more than 10 linked saccharide units (polysaccharides). Because their chemical structures are much larger and more complicated than those of sugars, starch and fiber are called complex carbohydrates. They do not taste sweet.

Monosaccharides

Monosaccharides consist of single saccharide (sugar) units. They form the building blocks of more complex carbohydrates. Three types of monosaccharides are significant in human nutrition, and all have the same basic hexagonal structure. The arrangement of the atoms that form the projecting side branches determines the type of sugar. Glucose (which has the molecular structure illustrated here) is the primary breakdown product of all other carbohydrates you eat. Glucose also occurs naturally in some fruits and plant juices. Fructose is present in some fruits and vegetables and in honey. Galactose does not occur in a free state but is one of the two sugar units that form lactose.

- Carbon
- Oxygen
- Hydrogen

Disaccharides

These double-unit sugars are formed when two simple sugars are bonded together by oxygen. A well-known disaccharide is sucrose (shown at right). Sucrose – ordinary table sugar – is a chemical combination of glucose and fructose. It is widely used as a sweetener in processed foods. Other disaccharides include lactose, found only in milk, and maltose, which is produced by the breakdown of starch and is also found in grains.

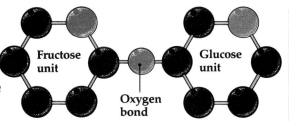
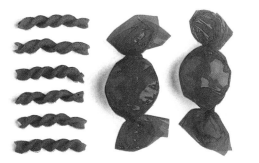

Fructose unit

Glucose unit

Oxygen bond

STRUCTURE OF STARCH

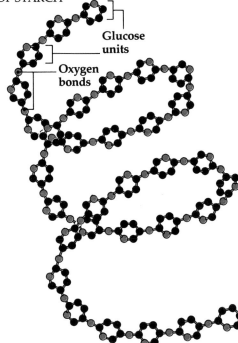

Glucose units

Oxygen bonds

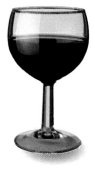

Polysaccharides

Under certain conditions, monosaccharides (most often glucose) link to form long chains of sugar units called polysaccharides. These chains can fold into compact structures that make them ideal as storage carbohydrates.

Starch, which consists of chains forming a helix shape (left), is the storage carbohydrate of plants. It is found in grains, vegetables, and fruits. Cellulose is also a polysaccharide but, unlike starch, the chains are straight and linked in a parallel fashion. This makes cellulose – insoluble fiber – impossible for our digestive enzymes to break down.

THE VALUE OF CARBO-HYDRATES

Try to obtain 55 to 60 percent of your energy from carbohydrates. While all sugars and starches provide about 4 kilocalories per gram, they are not equal nutritionally. Sucrose, whether eaten as pure sugar or as an additive, provides what is often called "empty calories." Food sources of unrefined carbohydrates, such as dried peas and beans, whole-grain products, and fresh fruit, contain vitamins, minerals, and fiber. Make an effort to eat the bulk of your carbohydrates in unrefined forms rather than in the form of processed foods.

IS ALCOHOL A FOOD?

The alcohol in beer, wine, and hard liquor provides some energy (7 kilocalories per gram of pure alcohol). Some alcoholic beverages contain additional calories in the form of carbohydrates such as maltose and sucrose (about 4 kilocalories per gram). Beer and wine also contain insignificant amounts of vitamins, minerals, and protein. Hard liquor contains no other nutrients. If a consistently large part of a person's energy requirements is provided by alcohol, malnutrition will soon occur.

The energy constituents of some alcoholic drinks

Jigger of hard liquor (1.5 fluid ounces, 80 proof)

Glass of beer (12 fluid ounces, 4.5% alcohol)

Glass of wine (3.5 fluid ounces, 12.2% alcohol)

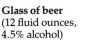

g = gram
kcal = kilocalorie

Ethyl alcohol 14 g
Carbohydrate 0 g
Total energy 97 kcal

Ethyl alcohol 11.7 g
Protein 1.1 g
Carbohydrate 13.7 g
Total energy 151 kcal

Ethyl alcohol 10.1 g
Carbohydrate 4.3 g
Total energy 87 kcal

CALORIES

The unit of food energy is the calorie (the amount of energy required to heat 1 milliliter of water 1°C). However, 1 calorie represents an extremely small amount of energy. The "calorie" that we are all familiar with refers to a kilocalorie (1,000 calories), which is also called a Calorie with a capital C. Food energy values in this book are given in kilocalories – the same as the calorie of popular usage.

To be used by your body, all carbohydrates must first be broken down into monosaccharides – glucose, fructose, and galactose – in the stomach and intestines (see THE DIGESTIVE PROCESS on page 44). These simple sugars are then absorbed into the bloodstream and can be used in various ways (see HOW THE BODY USES SUGARS FROM FOOD, at left). Excess glucose is converted into fatty acids and stored as fat as a longer-term energy source.

FATS

Fats, like carbohydrates, are used by your body primarily as an energy source. However, fats provide the energy in a more concentrated form – about 9 kilocalories per gram instead of the 4 kilocalories per gram provided by carbohydrates. Fats can be grouped into the "visible" and "invisible" types. Visible fats are apparent in butter, lard, margarine, and oils. Invisible fats are found in meat, poultry, fish, dairy products, eggs, nuts, legumes, and chocolate. In 1985, the average American consumed 25 pounds of all types of fat. Fats contribute significantly to the texture and palatability of the foods we eat. Fats fall into a variety of groups, including triglycerides and sterols (such as cholesterol).

The structure of a fat
Most naturally occurring fats are triglycerides similar to the one illustrated below. Triglycerides consist of three fatty acids and one molecule of glycerol linked by oxygen bonds.

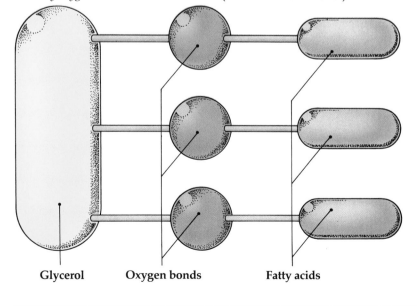

Glycerol   **Oxygen bonds**   **Fatty acids**

THE TRANSPORT OF FATS IN THE BLOOD

Fats are carried in the bloodstream bound to protein, forming particles called lipoproteins. Lipoproteins are classified according to the amount of protein they contain – the higher the proportion of protein, the greater the density. Each type of lipoprotein has a different role to play.

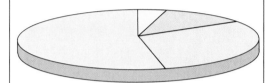

Very low-density lipoproteins (VLDLs)
These lipoproteins contain a large percentage of triglycerides, which are used by the body for energy or are stored as fat. VLDLs convert into low-density lipoproteins.

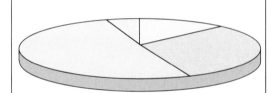

Low-density lipoproteins (LDLs)
LDLs contain a large percentage of cholesterol, which is used by cells for essential bodily functions. A high level of cholesterol carried in the blood in the form of LDLs is associated with an increased risk of atherosclerosis and heart disease.

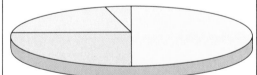

High-density lipoproteins (HDLs)
HDLs, like LDLs, also contain a large percentage of cholesterol, but they have a different job. HDLs remove cholesterol from the tissues and transport it to the liver for excretion. Because HDLs help rid the body of cholesterol, a high ratio of HDLs to LDLs seems to protect against heart disease.

☐ Protein   ☐ Cholesterol

☐ Phospholipid   ☐ Triglycerides

The composition of fats

Most of the fats in food are triglycerides, although some foods also contain small amounts of cholesterol. Triglycerides are a combination of three fatty acids with glycerol. The differences in fats result largely from the fatty acids involved.

How your body uses fats

Fats in the food you eat are dissolved in the intestine by the action of bile salts. The triglycerides are split into glycerol and fatty acids, which enter the wall of the intestine. There they are reconstituted into triglycerides, which are absorbed via the lymphatic system and carried to the bloodstream. The fat-soluble vitamins A, D, E, and K are absorbed at the same time as the fatty acids. Cholesterol does not need to be broken down before being absorbed into the lymphatic system.

SATURATED AND UNSATURATED FAT

All fats and oils found in food contain a mixture of saturated, monounsaturated, and polyunsaturated fatty acids in differing proportions. In general, animal and dairy fats, which remain solid at room temperature and are called hard fats, are a concentrated source of saturated fatty acids. Vegetable fats and oils (with the exception of coconut, palm, and palm kernel oils) contain larger amounts of unsaturated fatty acids and are liquid at room temperature. Of the vegetable oils, olive, canola, and peanut oil are rich in monounsaturated fatty acids.

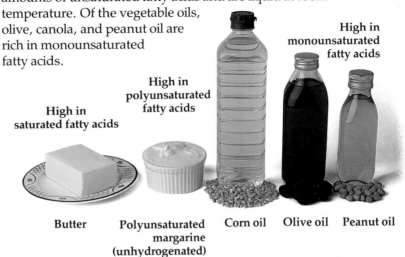

High in saturated fatty acids

High in polyunsaturated fatty acids

High in monounsaturated fatty acids

Butter **Polyunsaturated margarine (unhydrogenated)** **Corn oil** **Olive oil** **Peanut oil**

HOW NUTRIENTS PROVIDE ENERGY FOR CELLS

All body cells need a source of energy to function. Whatever the type of cell, its activities are powered by the splitting of a high-energy phosphate bond. This bond is formed using energy released by a complicated sequence of chemical reactions known as the Krebs cycle. The Krebs cycle takes place inside every cell of your body and is fueled by the breakdown products of the food you eat.

1 Glucose and fatty acids are the basic chemicals used in the Krebs cycle to produce energy. If there are insufficient amounts of these chemicals, amino acids may be used. Oxygen combines with the products of the Krebs cycle in a separate process.

2 The chemical adenosine triphosphate (ATP), present in all body cells, is split to release energy. In the process, ATP is converted to adenosine diphosphate (ADP). This chemical is continuously re-formed into ATP by energy released from food fuel (glucose and fat) during the Krebs cycle.

3 During the Krebs cycle, carbon dioxide is formed. Carbon dioxide is a waste product and is eliminated through the lungs and kidneys.

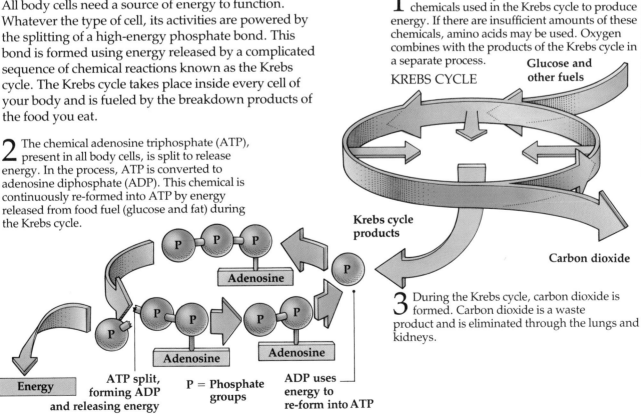

KREBS CYCLE

Glucose and other fuels

Krebs cycle products

Carbon dioxide

Energy   **ATP split, forming ADP and releasing energy**   **P = Phosphate groups**   **ADP uses energy to re-form into ATP**

Adenosine

Adenosine   Adenosine

PROTEIN SOURCES

The proteins contained in foods of animal origin are called complete proteins because they contain all the essential amino acids in approximately the same proportions as needed by the body. Proteins from plant sources, such as grains, legumes, and nuts, are called partially complete proteins because they are deficient in one or more essential amino acids. For this reason, animal proteins are generally considered superior to plant proteins. However, the amino acids deficient in one plant food are often present in another. By combining plant foods, as shown, it is possible to obtain the complete range of essential amino acids in balanced amounts.

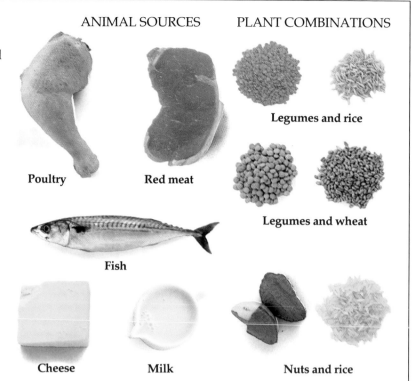

ANIMAL SOURCES

PLANT COMBINATIONS

Poultry

Red meat

Fish

Cheese

Milk

Legumes and rice

Legumes and wheat

Nuts and rice

IS MEAT THE IDEAL SOURCE OF PROTEIN?

Until recently, meat was considered an ideal food because of its protein content and many vitamins and minerals. But meat also contains animal fat. Eating too much meat can raise the level of cholesterol in your blood. When eaten to excess, meat can lead to an increased total calorie intake. It is now recommended that you eat from 4 to 6 ounces per day at the most. A more substantial proportion of your protein requirements may be chosen from low-fat dairy products, fish, and plant sources.

Inside your body, the fats you eat are used in a variety of ways.

◆ They are used as an immediate energy source. However, if there is more energy taken into the body (from food) than is expended during activity, the fat is deposited beneath the skin and around some internal organs.

◆ Cholesterol is an essential component of the walls of body cells and is required by the body for the formation of bile acids, which are secreted in the bile. Cholesterol, other sterols, and fatty acids may also be converted into vital hormones, vitamin D, phospholipids (which are essential components of body cells), and hormonelike substances such as prostaglandins.

PROTEINS

Proteins are large, complex molecules that consist of a string of basic building blocks, known as amino acids. Different amino acids can be linked in an almost infinite number of different ways to form different proteins.

Meat, poultry, fish, dairy products, eggs, cereals, legumes, and nuts contain substantial quantities of protein. Inside your body, proteins form the main structural elements of cells and tissues such as muscles, bones, connective tissues, and the walls of hollow organs. This makes proteins indispensable to growth, functioning, and repair. In addition, all the enzymes that regulate chemical reactions in your body are proteins.

During digestion, the proteins in food are broken down, first into polypeptides and peptides (short lengths of amino acids), and then into individual amino acids. The amino acids are absorbed into the bloodstream and distributed throughout the body, where they can be linked again into the specific structural proteins and enzymes needed by different body cells and tissues. If the energy available from carbohydrates and fats in the diet is not sufficient to meet demands, amino acids can also be converted into glucose or fatty acids and used as an energy source. However, since amino acids are not efficiently used for energy, and are important for maintaining tissue structure, they are used for energy only as a last resort.

The protein quality of foods

A total of 20 different amino acids is required to make proteins for the body. Of these, eight (known as essential amino acids) must be supplied in ready-made form by foods you eat. Others (known as nonessential amino acids) can be synthesized by the body itself as the need arises.

The nutritional value of a protein, which may be complete or incomplete, is judged by its ability to provide the body with essential amino acids (see PROTEIN SOURCES, at left).

Protein breakdown and synthesis
The proteins in food are different from those needed by body cells, but food proteins consist of the same amino acid building blocks. The diagram below shows how amino acids are released from food protein during digestion, then built up into new proteins in body cells.

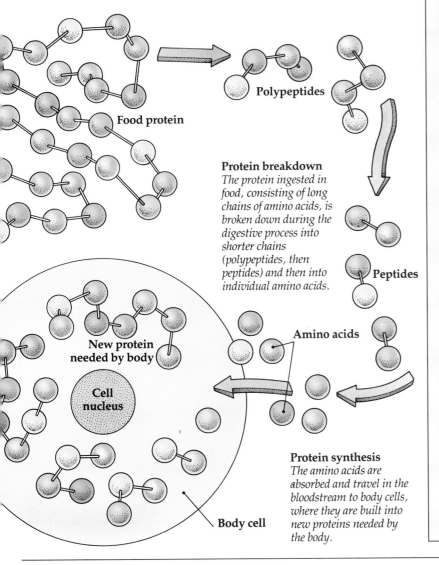

Food protein

Polypeptides

Protein breakdown
The protein ingested in food, consisting of long chains of amino acids, is broken down during the digestive process into shorter chains (polypeptides, then peptides) and then into individual amino acids.

Peptides

Amino acids

New protein needed by body

Cell nucleus

Body cell

Protein synthesis
The amino acids are absorbed and travel in the bloodstream to body cells, where they are built into new proteins needed by the body.

ASK YOUR DOCTOR FOOD FOR ENERGY AND GROWTH

Q I have read that fat is bad for us. Does that mean all kinds of fat – no matter what type?

A No. The Surgeon General in 1988 advised a reduction in the total amount of all fat in the diet – but particularly in the amount of saturated fats (those contained in meats, butter, lard, or tropical oils) – as a means of reducing the risk of heart disease. Unsaturated fats (contained in corn oil, olive oil, and other vegetable oils), when consumed in small amounts, may protect against heart disease. However, all fats contain between 100 and 120 kilocalories a tablespoon and should be consumed in moderation.

Q I love popcorn and have heard that it is a healthy, low-calorie snack. Is this true?

A Yes – if you prepare it correctly. One cup of plain, air-popped popcorn contains 23 kilocalories, less than 1 gram of fat, and only a trace of sodium. Popcorn also is a rich source of complex carbohydrates and fiber. However, if you choose to make popcorn with salt and oil or prepare microwave popcorn, the fat and sodium content can rise dramatically.

Q I have heard that many people eat more protein than they really need. Is this true?

A Excess protein generally causes problems only in people who have liver or kidney disease. The dietary guidelines recommend eating 4 to 6 ounces of protein a day. You can substitute 1 egg white, one half cup of cooked beans, or 2 tablespoons of peanut butter for 1 ounce of meat.

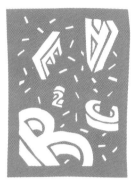

VITAMINS AND MINERALS

VITAMINS AND MINERALS are vital to the healthy functioning of your body. They are essential for growth, energy production, vitality, and general well-being. Most vitamins, and all minerals, must be provided directly by the food you eat because your body cannot manufacture them from other substances in food.

FAT- OR WATER-SOLUBLE VITAMINS

Vitamins A, D, E, and K are fat soluble; they are found in fat- or oil-containing foods. Fat-soluble vitamins are stored in the liver or in fatty tissue; an excess may be toxic. The B-complex vitamins and vitamin C are water soluble. Any excess is usually excreted via the urine.

This section reviews what vitamins and minerals are, what they do for your body, and what foods they are found in. It does not address daily requirements or the groups of people who may benefit from vitamin and mineral supplements. These issues are covered in VITAMIN AND MINERAL REQUIREMENTS on page 66. Specific vitamin and mineral deficiency diseases are addressed in VITAMIN AND MINERAL DEFICIENCIES on page 120.

Strictly, vitamins are substances that
♦ are essential for body functioning
♦ cannot be made by the body
♦ are required in small amounts
♦ if absent from the diet can lead to a recognized deficiency disease, such as scurvy or rickets.

In practice, although 13 "true" vitamins are recognized, one of these (vitamin D) can be made by human cells, another (niacin) can be made in the body from an amino acid, and two others (vitamin K and biotin) can be produced by bacteria in the colon, though not in sufficient quantity to meet needs.

Minerals are simple chemical elements, none of which can be synthesized by the body. A total of 16 are known to be essential.

WHAT ARE VITAMINS?

Vitamins have complex molecular structures, consisting mainly of the elements hydrogen, carbon, oxygen, and nitrogen. The structures of four different vitamins – two water soluble (B_6 and C) and two fat soluble (A and D) – are shown below. Vitamins are present in varying amounts in nearly all foods. Some vitamins (such as vitamin B_{12}) are found only or mainly in foods of animal origin, while others (such as vitamin E) are found primarily in vegetables.

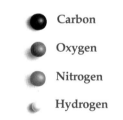

● Carbon
● Oxygen
● Nitrogen
◖ Hydrogen

GREEN LEAFY VEGETABLES
Green leafy vegetables are a good source of vitamin A, folic acid, vitamin C, and vitamin K. They also contain the minerals iron, magnesium, and potassium. Greens and broccoli are also sources of calcium.

OILY FISH
Fish with a high fat content such as tuna and salmon are a good source of vitamin B_6 and some contain vitamin D. These fish also contain iodine and selenium.

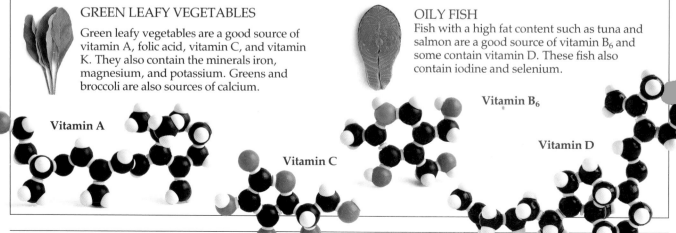

Vitamin A

Vitamin C

Vitamin B_6

Vitamin D

HOW YOUR BODY USES VITAMINS AND MINERALS

Vitamins and minerals are used in different ways by different parts of your body. Most are required throughout the body for general functioning, growth, and repair, but some have more specific roles; the major ones are shown below. Some vitamins and minerals are stored in your body for longer periods than others. However, without a regular supply, the body will eventually fail to function properly. There is significant interaction between vitamins and minerals; a deficiency or excess of one affects the others.

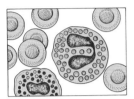

Blood cell formation and functioning
Vitamin B$_6$
Vitamin B$_{12}$
Folic acid
Vitamin E
Copper
Iron

Blood clotting
Vitamin K
Calcium

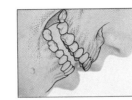

Healthy teeth
Vitamin C
Vitamin D
Calcium
Phosphorus
Fluorine
Magnesium

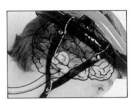

Nervous system functioning
Thiamine
Vitamin B$_6$
Vitamin B$_{12}$
Vitamin E
Biotin
Calcium
Potassium
Sodium
Magnesium

Muscle functioning
Thiamine
Calcium
Magnesium
Potassium
Sodium

Energy production
Thiamine
Riboflavin
Niacin
Pantothenic acid
Biotin
Calcium
Chromium
Copper
Iodine
Iron
Magnesium
Phosphorus
Potassium

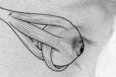

Healthy eyes
Vitamin A
Zinc

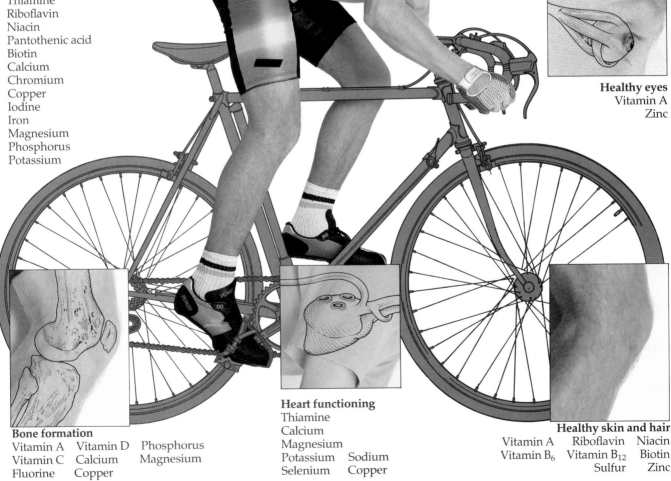

Bone formation

Vitamin A	Vitamin D	Phosphorus
Vitamin C	Calcium	Magnesium
Fluorine	Copper	

Heart functioning

Thiamine	
Calcium	
Magnesium	
Potassium	Sodium
Selenium	Copper

Healthy skin and hair

Vitamin A	Riboflavin	Niacin
Vitamin B$_6$	Vitamin B$_{12}$	Biotin
	Sulfur	Zinc

VITAMINS

Researchers studying nutritional deficiency diseases made the early discoveries about vitamins. Very little was known about the chemical structure of vitamins, and it was difficult to assign them a scientific name. Vitamins were first separated as fat-soluble A and water-soluble B, based on their ability to dissolve in either oil or water. Further study revealed that each group was made up of a combination of several substances, which were labeled sequentially by letters of the alphabet.

The common vitamins known today include A, the B-complex group, C, D, E, and K. The requirement for each of these vitamins in the human diet has been proven.

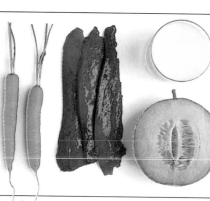

Functions
◆ keeps the surfaces of the corneas healthy
◆ essential for healthy skin, hair, and organ linings
◆ important for bone formation

Sources
◆ calf liver
◆ fortified milk products
◆ carrots
◆ dark green leafy vegetables
◆ eggs
◆ cantaloupes
◆ oranges
◆ oily fish
◆ apricots

VITAMIN A

Vitamin A, the most active form of which is known as retinol, is a fat-soluble vitamin. Vitamin A is found in a stored form in foods of animal origin. Beta-carotene, which converts to vitamin A in the intestine and liver, is present in yellow-orange and dark green vegetables and fruits.

B-COMPLEX VITAMINS

The B-complex vitamins are a group of closely related water-soluble substances that often occur together in foods of animal and plant origin. The B-complex vitamins include thiamine, riboflavin, niacin, vitamin B_6, folic acid, pantothenic acid, and biotin. Vitamin B_{12} is not usually considered part of the B-complex vitamins. Because the B-complex vitamins are not stored in the body for any length of time, a diet containing insufficient amounts can lead to deficiency symptoms within a few months. The B-complex vitamins work in unison to perform their functions, which are described below and opposite. The B-complex vitamins also assist enzymes, which are proteins that mediate the breakdown, synthesis, or interconversion of substances in the body.

Functions
◆ acts as a coenzyme, helping to convert glucose into energy
◆ essential for the function of the nervous system and muscles, including the heart muscle

Sources
◆ pork
◆ whole grains and grain products and fortified cereals and breads
◆ organ meats
◆ peas
◆ eggs
◆ potatoes
◆ fish
◆ dairy products

THIAMINE

Thiamine, also known as vitamin B_1, is a water-soluble vitamin. It is found in many animal and plant foods, ham and peas being particularly good sources. Thiamine is necessary for the steady and continuous release of energy from glucose in body cells, especially in muscles and nerves.

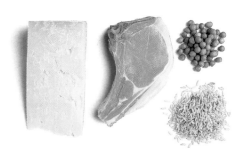

RIBOFLAVIN

Riboflavin, also known as vitamin B_2, is a water-soluble vitamin found in many animal and plant foods. Riboflavin is essential to the activity of many enzymes involved in the release of energy from proteins, carbohydrates, and fats in cells. It also helps maintain the mucous membranes.

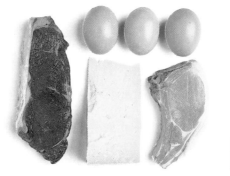

Functions
◆ necessary for the release of energy from carbohydrates, fats, and proteins
◆ maintains healthy skin

Sources
◆ milk
◆ liver
◆ cheese
◆ green leafy vegetables
◆ eggs
◆ meats
◆ other vegetables
◆ fruits
◆ nuts
◆ peas and beans

NIACIN

Niacin, also known as vitamin B_3, has two forms, nicotinic acid and nicotinamide. It is essential for the utilization of energy from food. Niacin is found in many animal and plant foods, and the body can manufacture its own niacin using the amino acid tryptophan. The diet usually needs to contain some nicotinic acid or nicotinamide to supply the daily requirements.

Functions

◆ necessary for the release of energy from nutrients such as glucose and fats
◆ essential for the synthesis of many important substances in the body, including some hormones
◆ maintains healthy skin

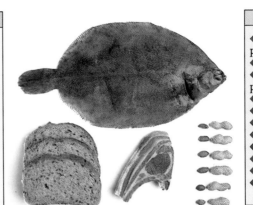

Sources

◆ meats and poultry
◆ fish
◆ whole-grain products
◆ liver
◆ peanuts
◆ cheese
◆ peas and beans
◆ potatoes
◆ milk
◆ eggs
◆ tuna

VITAMIN B_6

Vitamin B_6, also known as pyridoxine, is a water-soluble vitamin. It is actually a group of closely related substances – pyridoxine, pyridoxal, and pyridoxamine – that function together. Among other roles, vitamin B_6 regulates the synthesis of proteins from amino acids.

Functions

◆ necessary for hemoglobin formation
◆ required to help regulate the function of cells in the nervous system
◆ maintains healthy skin

Sources

◆ meats and poultry
◆ fish
◆ liver
◆ whole-grain products
◆ bananas
◆ most fruits and vegetables
◆ eggs
◆ dairy products

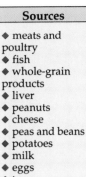

Functions

◆ required for growth and repair of cells
◆ essential for formation of red and white blood cells

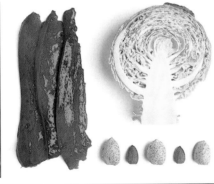

Sources

◆ green leafy vegetables
◆ organ meats
◆ nonleafy vegetables
◆ whole-wheat bread
◆ nuts
◆ mushrooms
◆ peas and beans

FOLIC ACID

Folic acid, sometimes called vitamin M, is a water-soluble vitamin and a member of the B-complex vitamin group. Its major functions are to promote the production of proteins and of RNA and DNA, the genetic material of all cells. Folic acid also works with vitamin B_{12} to form red blood cells.

Functions

◆ essential for formation of rapidly growing cells, including red and white blood cells in bone marrow, cells of the intestinal lining, and hair follicles
◆ maintains healthy nervous system

Sources

◆ liver
◆ beef
◆ pork
◆ lamb
◆ poultry
◆ fish
◆ milk and milk products
◆ eggs
◆ oysters
◆ yeast

VITAMIN B_{12}

Vitamin B_{12} is also known as cyanocobalamin (a synthetic form). It contains the mineral cobalt and is water soluble. Vitamin B_{12} is made by bacteria. It is absorbed into the tissues of ruminating animals (such as cows) or omnivorous animals, both of which ingest bacteria in their food. Foods of animal origin are the only significant sources of vitamin B_{12}. Vitamin B_{12} helps in the formation of red blood cells, aids in the functioning of the nervous system, and assists in the construction of genetic material.

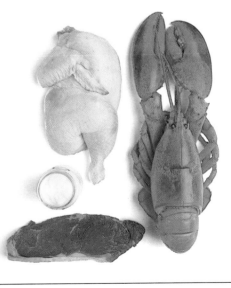

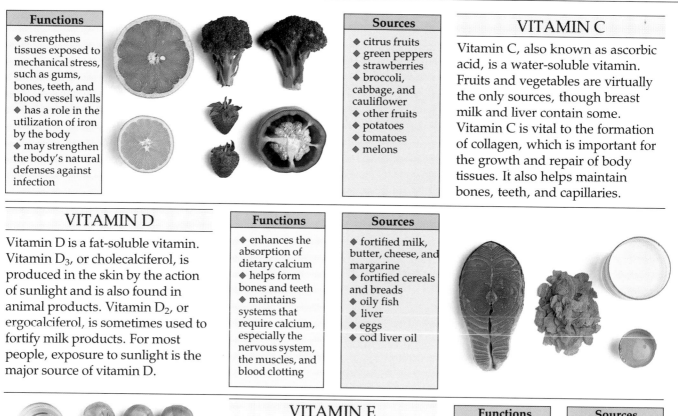

Functions

◆ strengthens tissues exposed to mechanical stress, such as gums, bones, teeth, and blood vessel walls
◆ has a role in the utilization of iron by the body
◆ may strengthen the body's natural defenses against infection

Sources

◆ citrus fruits
◆ green peppers
◆ strawberries
◆ broccoli, cabbage, and cauliflower
◆ other fruits
◆ potatoes
◆ tomatoes
◆ melons

VITAMIN C

Vitamin C, also known as ascorbic acid, is a water-soluble vitamin. Fruits and vegetables are virtually the only sources, though breast milk and liver contain some. Vitamin C is vital to the formation of collagen, which is important for the growth and repair of body tissues. It also helps maintain bones, teeth, and capillaries.

VITAMIN D

Vitamin D is a fat-soluble vitamin. Vitamin D_3, or cholecalciferol, is produced in the skin by the action of sunlight and is also found in animal products. Vitamin D_2, or ergocalciferol, is sometimes used to fortify milk products. For most people, exposure to sunlight is the major source of vitamin D.

Functions

◆ enhances the absorption of dietary calcium
◆ helps form bones and teeth
◆ maintains systems that require calcium, especially the nervous system, the muscles, and blood clotting

Sources

◆ fortified milk, butter, cheese, and margarine
◆ fortified cereals and breads
◆ oily fish
◆ liver
◆ eggs
◆ cod liver oil

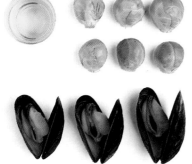

VITAMIN E

Vitamin E, also called tocopherol, is a fat-soluble vitamin. It helps prevent certain oxidation reactions in the body, protecting tissues against oxidizing substances that are thought to contribute to degenerative changes in organs. Rich sources include vegetable oils, whole-grain cereals, and dried beans.

Functions

◆ protects cell membranes from damage
◆ plays a part in red blood cell formation and protection of red blood cells from damage

Sources

◆ vegetable oils
◆ margarine
◆ eggs
◆ fish
◆ green leafy vegetables
◆ whole-grain products
◆ dried beans

Functions

◆ essential for the formation in the liver of substances that promote blood clotting
◆ important for calcium metabolism in bone

VITAMIN K

Vitamin K is a fat-soluble vitamin that is necessary for normal blood clotting. There are two natural forms, K_1 and K_2. K_1 is found in foods of plant origin. K_2 can be formed by bacteria in the intestines. K_3, also called menadione, is synthetic.

Sources

◆ green leafy vegetables
◆ pork liver
◆ cauliflower
◆ grain products
◆ potatoes
◆ fruits
◆ milk and eggs
◆ cheese
◆ cabbage

PANTOTHENIC ACID AND BIOTIN

◆ **Pantothenic acid** is needed for the release of energy from food and for the production of some hormones and other substances. It is found in both animal and plant foods.
◆ **Biotin** aids the action of enzymes involved in the synthesis of substances in cells. It is fairly widely distributed in foods; small amounts can also be made by intestinal bacteria.

FALSE VITAMINS

The following substances are not vitamins, either because there is no evidence that they are needed by the body or because they can be made in the body:
◆ orotic acid
◆ pangamic acid
◆ amygdalin
◆ choline
◆ inositol
◆ carnitine
◆ para-aminobenzoic acid (PABA)
◆ bioflavonoid complex

MINERALS

In addition to the elements carbon, oxygen, hydrogen, and nitrogen, which are present in large amounts in nutrients and in the body, your diet must provide several other chemical elements, called minerals. Minerals are an essential part of your body's functioning. The best way to get the minerals you need in the correct amounts is by eating the widest possible variety of foods. The major minerals, which are needed in relatively large quantities, are calcium, phosphorus, sodium, potassium, magnesium, chlorine, and sulfur. The remaining minerals – sometimes called essential trace elements – are needed in much smaller amounts. They include iron, copper, fluorine, iodine, selenium, zinc, chromium, cobalt, manganese, and molybdenum. Several other elements are candidates for essential trace element status even though little is known about their functions in the body.

MINERAL NEEDS

The minerals you need are listed in the box ARE YOU GETTING ENOUGH MINERALS? on page 70. There is no evidence that any mineral taken in greater quantities than recommended improves health. Many megadoses are toxic or interfere with the absorption and/ or function of other essential minerals.

MINERAL DEFICIENCIES

Deficiencies of the minerals calcium and iron are common. Deficiencies of other minerals can also occur but only if the diet is highly restricted or consists primarily of highly processed foods. Mineral deficiencies are addressed under VITAMIN AND MINERAL DEFICIENCIES on page 120.

CALCIUM

There is more calcium in your body than any other mineral. You lose calcium continuously, so an adequate intake is necessary throughout life. Children, adolescents, and young adults need a particularly high intake. Calcium requirements also increase during pregnancy and lactation. These are times when women have an increased loss of calcium and protein from bones, making them much more likely than men to get osteoporosis. An adequate calcium intake along with weight-bearing exercise, such as brisk walking, can retard the loss of bone density.

Functions
◆ needed to form and maintain healthy bones and teeth
◆ essential for contraction of muscles, including the heart
◆ needed for efficient conduction of impulses along nerves
◆ aids blood clotting
◆ required for activity of several enzymes required by all cells
◆ maintains tight junctions between cells and tissues

Sources
◆ milk and dairy products
◆ fish with edible bones, such as sardines or canned salmon
◆ green leafy vegetables
◆ eggs
◆ dried peas and beans
◆ nuts and seeds
◆ oysters and shrimp
◆ citrus fruits

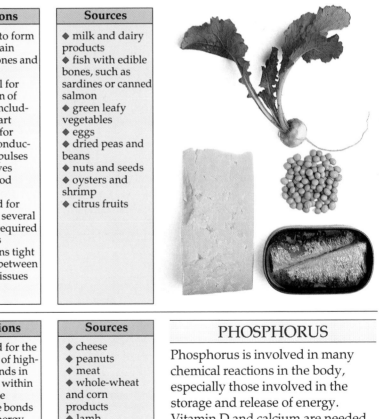

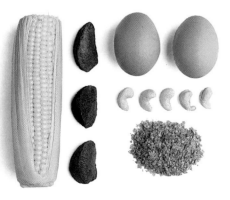

Functions
◆ required for the formation of high-energy bonds in molecules within cells. These phosphate bonds transfer energy from ingested fat, carbohydrate, and protein to the cell
◆ necessary for the structure of crystals in bones and teeth

Sources
◆ cheese
◆ peanuts
◆ meat
◆ whole-wheat and corn products
◆ lamb
◆ fish
◆ milk
◆ rice
◆ nuts
◆ eggs
◆ dried peas and beans

PHOSPHORUS

Phosphorus is involved in many chemical reactions in the body, especially those involved in the storage and release of energy. Vitamin D and calcium are needed in conjunction with phosphorus for development and maintenance of the skeleton. Phosphorus is found in many foods. In general, if your protein intake is adequate, your phosphorus intake will be too.

SODIUM

Sodium is one of the most important substances in body fluids. It is involved primarily with the maintenance of the body's water balance and is essential for the functioning of nerves and muscles. Sodium is found in many naturally occurring foods and is added to many processed foods.

Functions
◆ regulates water balance
◆ essential to the generation of electrical charges involved in muscle contraction and nerve transmission
◆ involved in control of heart rhythms

Sources
◆ smoked, cured, or pickled meats and fish
◆ pickled vegetables
◆ canned soups
◆ tomato juice
◆ olives
◆ cheese
◆ table salt

POTASSIUM

Potassium, in conjunction with sodium, is essential to the regulation of the body's water balance and to nerve and muscle function. Severe diarrhea or vomiting causes loss of potassium, as do certain kidney diseases and excessive use of diuretic drugs.

Functions
◆ essential to the generation of electrical charges involved in muscle contraction and nerve transmission
◆ a normal concentration maintains regular heart rhythm

Sources
◆ potatoes
◆ dried fruits
◆ nuts
◆ beans
◆ bananas
◆ green leafy vegetables
◆ fruits
◆ meat
◆ milk
◆ fish

MAGNESIUM

More than half the magnesium in your body is found in your bones. Magnesium is also essential for nerve and muscle function. Severe deficiency is rare and is usually a result of excessive diarrhea or alcohol abuse. Marginal deficiency may be common.

Functions
◆ important for bone and tooth structure
◆ essential to the activity of many body enzymes
◆ needed for nerve impulse transmission
◆ needed for muscle function

Sources
◆ nuts
◆ whole-grain cereals
◆ dark green vegetables
◆ clams and other seafood
◆ dairy products
◆ meats
◆ dried fruits
◆ hard water

IRON

Most of the iron in your body is present in hemoglobin and myoglobin, the oxygen-carrying pigments of blood and muscle. Iron from the hemoglobin in meat is better absorbed than iron from vegetables.

Functions
◆ necessary for formation of hemoglobin in red blood cells
◆ acts as oxygen reservoir in muscles
◆ essential to activity of some enzymes

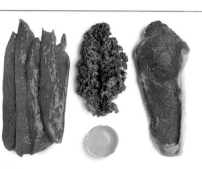

Sources
◆ liver
◆ red meat
◆ shellfish
◆ nuts
◆ egg yolk
◆ enriched breads, cereals, rice, and pasta
◆ some green leafy vegetables

COPPER

Copper takes part in many enzyme activities in the body. Except for certain genetic disorders, the body regulates the absorption of copper well. Disease due to deficiency is rare, but many people may have a marginal deficiency because they are not eating enough foods that contain copper.

Functions
◆ essential to the activity of many enzymes, including those involved in the formation of skin pigments and connective tissues
◆ helps incorporate iron into hemoglobin

Sources
◆ organ meats
◆ crustaceans and shellfish
◆ mushrooms
◆ nuts, beans, and peas
◆ whole-grain cereals and breads
◆ dried fruits
◆ grapes

Functions	Sources
◆ is incorporated into the crystal-line structure of, and thus strengthens, bones and teeth ◆ strengthens the mineral composition of tooth enamel	◆ fish and other seafood ◆ tea ◆ fluoridated drinking water

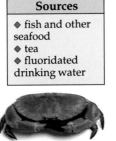

FLUORINE

Fluorine is needed to form strong, hard bones and teeth. The soil in which the food is grown is more important than the type of food itself. This is also true of some other trace elements, such as iodine and selenium. However, seafood is always rich in fluorine.

IODINE

You need iodine for the formation of thyroid hormones. Deficiency leads to enlargement of the thyroid gland, a condition called goiter. The best source is seafood. In noncoastal regions, iodized salt is a useful source.

Functions	Sources
◆ a component of thyroid hormones (produced by the thyroid gland), which control the rate of energy release in the body	◆ salt water fish ◆ shellfish ◆ iodized salt

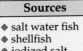

Functions	Sources
◆ helps protect cells and tissues from oxidation ◆ may protect against some cancers induced by oxidizing substances released in the body	◆ fish and shellfish ◆ meat ◆ whole-grain cereals ◆ dairy products

SELENIUM

Selenium, like vitamin E, functions as an antioxidant, which means that it protects against damage to cells and tissues by oxidation. The selenium content of foods varies according to its content in the soil from which the food originated.

ZINC

Zinc is a constituent of many enzymes needed for growth and energy production. The highest concentrations are found in your bones. While serious dietary deficiency of zinc is rare, marginal deficiency may be common.

Functions	Sources
◆ required for growth and energy production ◆ essential for testicular function, sperm formation ◆ helps heal wounds and maintains healthy skin and eyes	◆ oysters ◆ meat ◆ whole-grain cereals ◆ beans ◆ nuts ◆ eggs ◆ fish

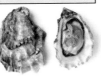

OTHER ESSENTIAL MINERALS

◆ **Chlorine** is usually associated with sodium, both in foods and in body fluids. The kidneys regulate chlorine to maintain water and acid-base balance.

◆ **Sulfur** is part of two amino acids that are used to build body proteins and is also present in the vitamins biotin and thiamine. Sulfur is found in all protein-containing foods.

◆ **Chromium** is needed to enhance the action of the hormone insulin in the utilization of glucose.

◆ **Cobalt** is not known to have any functions in the body except as part of vitamin B_{12}. Food sources are as for vitamin B_{12}.

◆ **Manganese** assists the action of many enzymes but is essential to the activity of few of them. Tea and most plant foods contain manganese.

◆ **Molybdenum** is part of the structure of several enzymes in the body. Meat, whole grains, peas, and beans are good food sources.

ASK YOUR DOCTOR VITAMINS AND MINERALS

Q If I were to get all my vitamins and minerals from a pill, could I stop eating?

A No. Vitamin and mineral supplements are not substitutes for food. They provide no energy and cannot replace protein, carbohydrates, fats, or water, which maintain tissues and organs.

Q My mother buys lots of vitamins and makes me take them too. I'm 18 and I'm leaving home next year to go to college. Should I spend my money on vitamins?

A The value of vitamin supplements is highly controversial. Your mother probably isn't doing herself – or you – any harm unless the dosages are well above the RDAs (check the label). Nutrients can be obtained in sufficient amounts in carefully chosen foods. If you go to college and eat a well-balanced, varied mixture of foods, you don't need the supplements.

Q Are there any nutrient deficiencies to which women are particularly prone?

A Iron and calcium deficiencies are most commonly experienced by women. Pregnant and breast-feeding women need more calcium. Losses of iron are particularly high during menstruation.

THE DIGESTIVE PROCESS

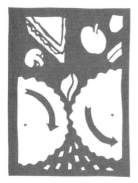

THE DIGESTIVE TRACT is a marvelously constructed, 30-foot-long, muscular organ that can open to the environment at both ends. Its function is to break down the food and drink we consume into proteins, carbohydrates, and fats and then into smaller, simpler forms so that they can pass into the bloodstream, the liver, and, ultimately, the body cells where they are needed.

1 Mouth and esophagus
Food is ground up and mixed with saliva. Saliva contains the enzyme amylase, which starts to break down starch. After the mixture has been swallowed, it is propelled down the esophagus.

3 Gallbladder
The gallbladder concentrates and stores bile, a substance produced by the liver to aid the digestion of fat.

4 Pancreas
Powerful enzymes secreted by the pancreas are essential to the breakdown of proteins, carbohydrates, and fats. Bicarbonate, which is also secreted, neutralizes the acidity produced by the hydrochloric acid in gastric secretions.

2 Stomach
The churning action of the stomach mixes the food with gastric juices secreted by the stomach wall. Gastric juices contain hydrochloric acid and enzymes, which begin to break down proteins and fats, and intrinsic factor, which later aids in the absorption of vitamin B_{12} from food through the wall of the small intestine. When the food has been reduced to a thick, souplike liquid (known as chyme), it passes into the duodenum at a regulated rate.

HOW LONG DOES IT TAKE?
The drawing shows the approximate time it takes for food to pass through each part of the digestive system. The length of time food spends in the stomach depends on the type of food eaten. Liquids pass through almost immediately.

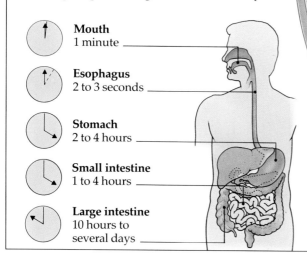

Mouth
1 minute

Esophagus
2 to 3 seconds

Stomach
2 to 4 hours

Small intestine
1 to 4 hours

Large intestine
10 hours to several days

5 Duodenum
As soon as food enters the duodenum, bile from the gallbladder and digestive juices from the pancreas are released and pour onto the now semiliquid food to continue the process of breaking it down.

6 Small intestine

It is here that the most important digestive processes take place. Intestinal juices secreted by the lining of the small intestine join bile and pancreatic juices to complete the breakdown of food. Nutrients are absorbed through small fingerlike projections called villi in the intestinal lining; they then pass into the bloodstream or the lymphatic ducts for utilization by the body, sometimes after further processing by the liver. Most water, vitamins, and minerals are also absorbed here. Any undigested material and remaining water pass into the large intestine.

Blood supply to small intestine
The specimen of the small intestine above shows the rich blood supply to its walls.

WHY DOESN'T THE STOMACH DIGEST ITSELF?

The enzymes and hydrochloric acid secreted by the stomach are powerful substances capable of eating into the stomach lining. However, the lining is not destroyed because the inside of the stomach is coated with special cells (see arrow) that secrete a protective mucus onto its surface.

7 Large intestine

Water and salt are absorbed through the walls of the large intestine. Remaining waste matter passes to the rectum for excretion.

Lining of large intestine
The image below shows the openings of mucus-secreting glands. Mucus provides lubrication for the passage of feces.

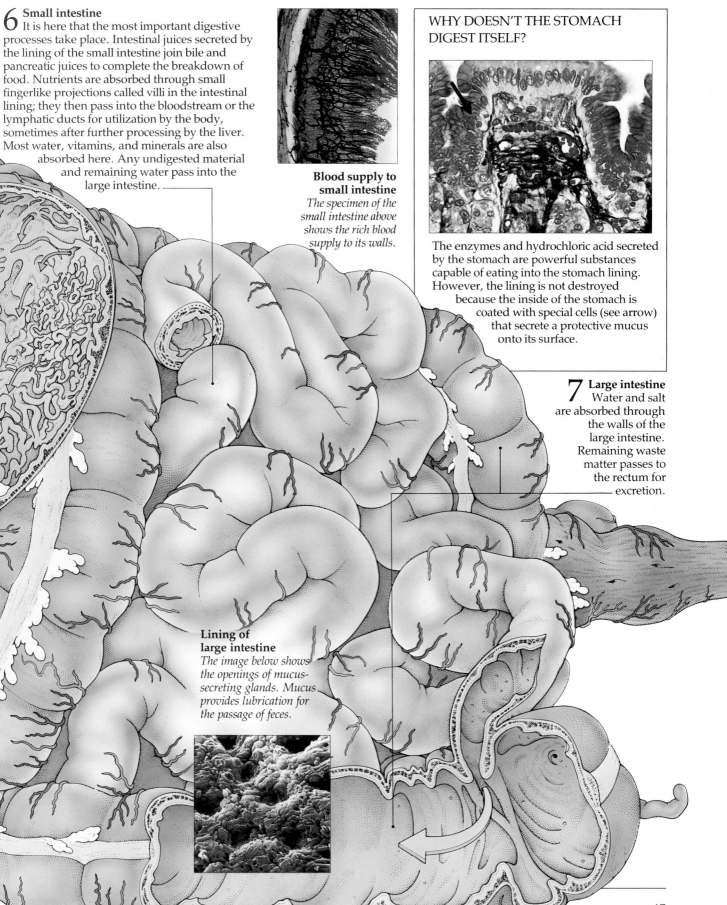

HOW FOOD IS BROKEN DOWN

Some constituents of our diet – water, salts, and all minerals and vitamins except vitamin B_{12} – can be absorbed directly into the body from the intestines. However, proteins, fats, and carbohydrates need to be broken down into smaller molecules before absorption can take place. Proteins are split into polypeptides, peptides, and amino acids. Carbohydrates are broken down into the simple sugars (monosaccharides) glucose, fructose, and galactose. Fats are partly split into fatty acids and glycerol.

IN THE MOUTH AND ESOPHAGUS

The enzyme amylase in saliva begins the breakdown of starch (one type of carbohydrate) by converting it into maltose (a sugar).

IN THE DUODENUM

Lipase (a pancreatic enzyme), with the help of bile salts (produced by the liver), splits fats into fatty acids and glycerol.

Amylase, secreted by the pancreas, splits starch into maltose and glucose.

Trypsin and chymotrypsin, secreted by the pancreas, split proteins into peptides and amino acids.

IN THE SMALL INTESTINE

Maltase, sucrase, and lactase (enzymes secreted by glands in the intestinal wall) break down maltose, sucrose, and lactose (types of double sugars known as disaccharides) into monosaccharides. Maltase converts maltose to glucose. Sucrase converts sucrose to glucose and fructose. Lactase converts lactose to glucose and galactose.

Peptidase, secreted by the intestinal wall, breaks large peptides into smaller peptides and amino acids.

IN THE STOMACH

Pepsin, which is secreted by the stomach lining, breaks down protein into peptides.

Lipase, also produced in the stomach, begins to break down fats.

The **hydrochloric acid** contained in gastric juice provides a suitable environment for the action of pepsin. Hydrochloric acid also destroys almost all of the bacteria that enter the body with food or water.

IN THE LARGE INTESTINE

The primary function of the large intestine is to absorb water from the undigested material arriving from the small intestine and compress it into semisolid feces ready for excretion.

Most of the nutrients are absorbed through the lining of the small intestine. The residue passes into the large intestine.

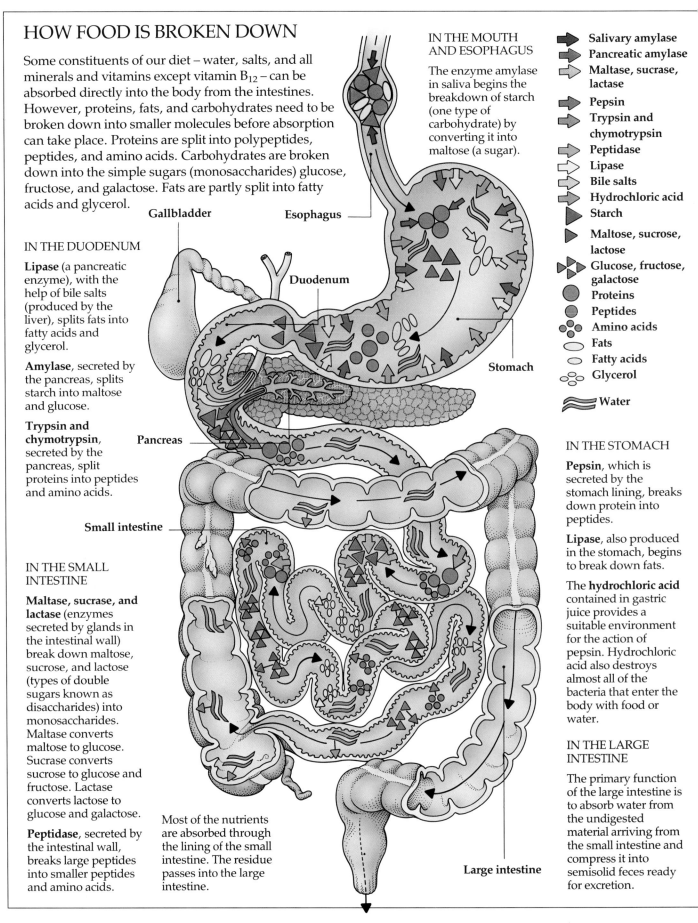

Legend:
- Salivary amylase
- Pancreatic amylase
- Maltase, sucrase, lactase
- Pepsin
- Trypsin and chymotrypsin
- Peptidase
- Lipase
- Bile salts
- Hydrochloric acid
- Starch
- Maltose, sucrose, lactose
- Glucose, fructose, galactose
- Proteins
- Peptides
- Amino acids
- Fats
- Fatty acids
- Glycerol
- Water

Labels: Gallbladder, Esophagus, Duodenum, Stomach, Pancreas, Small intestine, Large intestine

DIGESTION OF A PROTEIN

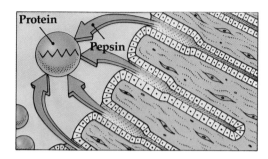

Splitting a protein into peptides
Glands in the stomach secrete the enzyme pepsin, which breaks down protein molecules into polypeptides. These are broken down into peptides.

Splitting peptides into amino acids
Enzymes produced in the pancreas pour into the small intestine. They join enzymes secreted by the intestinal walls to complete the breakdown of peptides into amino acids.

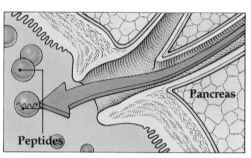

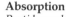

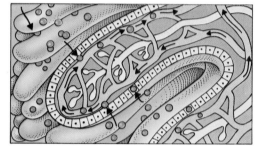

Absorption
Peptides and amino acids, along with some other nutrients, are absorbed through the tiny villi (see below) that line the intestinal walls. They then pass into the bloodstream.

ABSORPTION

Almost all absorption takes place through the walls of the small intestine, which are lined with millions of projections called villi. Villi give the small intestine a surface area about the size of a tennis court. Inside the villi are tiny blood vessels and lymph vessels called lacteals. Simple sugars, some peptides, and amino acids pass through the villi and are absorbed into the capillaries. From there they enter the intestinal veins and are carried to the liver for processing. As fatty acids and glycerol pass into the villi they recombine to form triglycerides, which are used as energy.

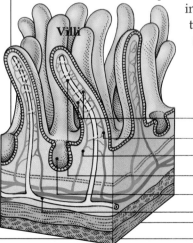

— Capillaries
— Vein
— Artery
— Lacteal
— Intestinal gland
— Lymph vessel

HUNGER AND APPETITE

The sensation of hunger occurs when the stomach is empty and the amount of certain nutrients, such as glucose, in the blood has reached a low level. Sensory receptors in the stomach and bloodstream detect these changes and signal centers in the brain concerned with the motivation to eat. These centers may also be affected by signals from the body's internal clocks. We tend to feel more hungry at those times of the day when we are accustomed to eating. The sensation of hunger includes an element of physical discomfort – the familiar gnawing sensation in the stomach – as well as feelings of weakness and, in some people, of increasing irritability.

Eating for pleasure

A simple model of eating behavior might state that we eat until uncomfortable sensations of hunger have been reduced (i.e., when the stomach has been filled and the level of nutrients in the bloodstream has been restored). In practice, the feeling of hunger is quickly satisfied, almost as soon as eating begins.

Clearly, we also eat for pleasure. Food, expressed in the dishes we prepare and serve, is an integral part of our lives. The pleasurable aspects of eating are embodied in the sensation of appetite and the sharing of meals with others. Other factors that contribute to appetite include the sight, smell, taste, and the anticipation of food, and the setting in which meals are eaten. Like hunger, appetite is a temporary phenomenon that gradually diminishes as food fills the stomach and the blood is replenished with nutrients. For most people, eating stops before the uncomfortable feelings of a bloated stomach supervene. However, the threshold at which satiety is reached varies among individuals and may be affected by factors such as habit, emotional state, size of stomach, previous eating behavior, and the degree to which a person's personality and psyche center around food and its consumption.

FIBER AND WATER

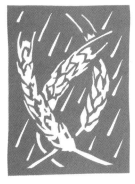

F IBER AND WATER are important constituents of food. Water is vital to life. About 55 to 65 percent of your body is made up of water, and many body functions require water. Although fiber cannot be absorbed by your body, it plays a vital role in the digestive process. By adding bulk to the feces, fiber encourages the efficient passage of waste products through the bowel and is thought by some experts to protect against a variety of diseases.

Dietary fiber consists of those parts of plant foods that cannot be broken down by enzymes in the human digestive tract. Most of the fiber we eat comes from the tough material in vegetables, the skin and flesh of fruits, and the husks of grains. Fiber plays a role in the maintenance of healthy bowel function. It also delays the body's absorption of refined sugars, thus modulating the rise in blood sugar after a meal.

TYPES OF FIBER

Fiber is not a single substance but a collection of substances. Some forms of fiber, known as insoluble fiber, pass through the intestine unchanged. Cellulose, hemicellulose, and lignins are insoluble fibers and are the primary fiber in such foods as the bran in whole-wheat bread and breakfast cereals and in beans

Fiber from foods
The table at right lists some common high-fiber foods. Almost all fruits and vegetables are good sources of fiber, although only a few are listed here. A sensible intake of dietary fiber is about 26 grams per day. It is best to obtain your fiber from a variety of food sources. Avoid increasing your fiber intake dramatically; a reduction in your body's ability to absorb minerals could result.

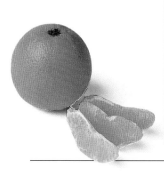

HIGH-FIBER FOODS	
FOOD	DIETARY FIBER per ounce (28 grams)
Unprocessed bran	12.3 grams
Dried apricots	7 grams
Prunes	4 grams
Almonds	4 grams
Raisins	2 grams
Whole-grain bread	2 grams
Dried beans	2 grams
Spinach or peas	2 grams
Peanut butter	2 grams
Broccoli or leeks	1 gram
Boiled lentils	1 gram
Apples, bananas, or strawberries	0.5 grams
Oranges or pears	0.4 grams

Structure of fiber
Cellulose (a type of soluble fiber) consists of chains of sugar molecules linked in a parallel fashion (shown below). Because human digestive enzymes are unable to break down such links, fiber cannot be absorbed by the body. The appearance of cellulose as seen under an electron microscope is shown at right.

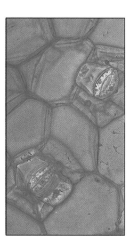

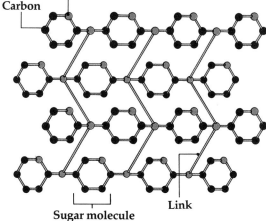

Oxygen

Carbon

Sugar molecule

Link

and peas. Other types, called soluble fiber, are acted on by bacteria in the colon (large intestine) and broken down into simpler components. Pectins and gums are examples of soluble fibers. Good sources of soluble fiber include rolled oats, dried beans, many fruits (such as apples), and green vegetables.

FIBER, HEALTH, AND DISEASE

A number of diseases, such as coronary heart disease, diabetes mellitus, cancer of the colon and rectum, diverticulosis, gallstones, and appendicitis, are common in Americans, but are rare in people who live in developing countries. Researchers have considered many environmental factors to account for these differences; among the more plausible are dietary differences. Fiber is a major component of the diets of rural populations in developing countries.

Digestive tract disease
Many of the valuable effects of fiber result from its remarkable ability to bind water during digestion. This ensures that the feces are soft and easy to pass and large enough to stretch the muscle and stimulate the contraction that propels them through the intestine.

Because it promotes bowel action and increases the frequency of elimination, fiber is an effective treatment for constipation. Diverticular disease, in which pouches form in the colon, is thought to be caused by raised pressure in the colon. Small, hard pieces of feces, called fecaliths, are known to block the appendix and cause appendicitis. The effort of expelling hard feces is thought to contribute to hemorrhoids. Each of these conditions can be ameliorated when a soft, formed stool can be passed regularly without straining. Dietary fiber is an important factor in achieving this.

Dietary fiber also binds simple sugars and regulates how quickly they are

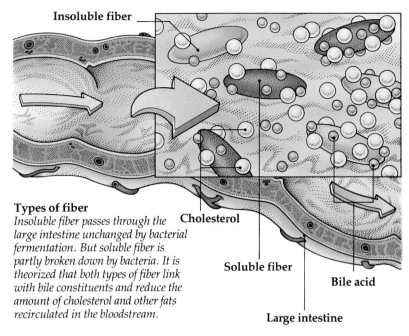

Insoluble fiber — **Cholesterol** — **Soluble fiber** — **Bile acid** — **Large intestine**

Types of fiber
Insoluble fiber passes through the large intestine unchanged by bacterial fermentation. But soluble fiber is partly broken down by bacteria. It is theorized that both types of fiber link with bile constituents and reduce the amount of cholesterol and other fats recirculated in the bloodstream.

HOW TO INCREASE YOUR INTAKE OF FIBER

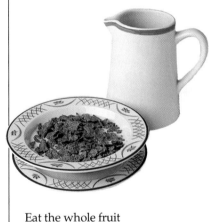
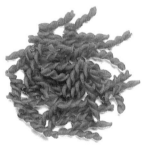

Eat more bran, whole-grain products (such as pasta and brown rice), and legumes. It's a good idea to start the day with a whole-grain breakfast cereal or whole-grain bread. Flour made from whole wheat contains three times as much dietary fiber as white flour, which is refined.

Eat the whole fruit rather than drinking a glass of fruit juice. One orange contains about six times as much fiber as a 4-ounce glass of orange juice.

Eat plenty of fruits and vegetables. Apples, grapefruits, brussels sprouts, broccoli, and pinto and navy beans are all good sources of soluble fiber.

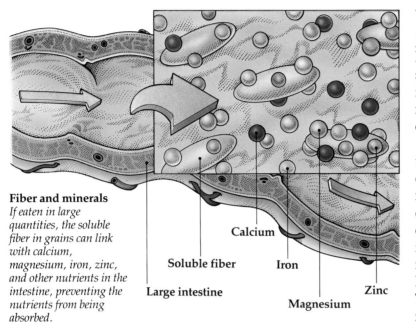

Fiber and minerals
If eaten in large quantities, the soluble fiber in grains can link with calcium, magnesium, iron, zinc, and other nutrients in the intestine, preventing the nutrients from being absorbed.

Calcium

Soluble fiber   Iron

Large intestine   Zinc

Magnesium

MINERAL DEFICIENCY

Fiber can bind important minerals such as calcium, magnesium, zinc, and iron in the intestine, making them unavailable for absorption by your body. However, you would need to consume large quantities of fiber – more than it would be possible to obtain from food alone – before decreased mineral absorption posed a health risk. Remember that fiber exists in a highly concentrated form in fiber supplements like unprocessed bran. Nutritionally vulnerable people, such as elderly people who have a low mineral intake, should be particularly careful when using these concentrated forms of fiber.

---

absorbed. This prevents blood sugar levels from rising sharply after a meal.

Fiber and artery disease

The relationship between dietary fiber and arterial diseases, such as atherosclerosis, is complex. It is theorized that both soluble and insoluble fiber are able to bind fats and constituents of bile (which contains cholesterol and bile acids derived from cholesterol) in the intestines, thus reducing the amount of fat and cholesterol that is recirculated in the bloodstream. This would be expected to lower the blood level of cholesterol, which is an important component of the plaques that are the main feature of atherosclerosis.

In practice, it is only the soluble fiber, such as pectins and guar gum found in apples and oats, that seems to have any cholesterol-lowering effect. The reasons for this effect are not clear. It may be that soluble fiber substitutes for the fats that would have been otherwise eaten. Some studies have shown that high cholesterol levels in the blood can be reduced by a high-fiber diet, especially if it contains soluble fiber. In people with normal cholesterol levels, the cholesterol-lowering effect is not as pronounced.

TOO MUCH FIBER

If a lack of dietary fiber is associated with so many disorders, should you eat as much fiber as possible? The answer is no. Too much fiber in your diet, as with too much of any nutrient, can cause problems.

While high-fiber diets are valuable in the treatment of chronic constipation, diverticulosis, and irritable colon, too much fiber can cause irritation of your digestive tract. Many people who embark on a high-fiber diet feel uncomfortable initially and experience abdominal cramps and an increase in flatulence. Increase your fiber intake gradually. The National Cancer Institute recommends a daily fiber intake of 26 grams.

If you rely on food sources for your fiber, it is difficult to take in too much; there are limits to the amount of high-fiber foods you can comfortably consume. The potential for ingesting too much fiber is increased if you use unprocessed bran or commercial fiber supplements. These products are highly concentrated sources of fiber.

WATER

Many bodily processes rely on water. If you lose more water than you take in, dehydration develops and body function slows. In a dehydrated state, it can become impossible for the body to regulate its temperature. In most cases, the thirst mechanism ensures that water losses from your body are matched by water intake. However, in a hot and dry climate you may need to drink more water than you think you do.

WATER BALANCE IN THE BODY

To prevent dehydration, the amount of water lost from the body must be matched by the intake. The illustration shows the average daily consumption and loss of water for an adult living in a temperate climate. The amount lost in sweat varies according to the climate and a person's level of activity. You must replace fluids lost through an increase in sweating. A marathon runner, for example, loses 8 to 10 pints (128 to 160 fluid ounces) of water during a race. It is extremely important for him or her to replace the lost fluid by drinking liquids along the way, since dehydration can make it impossible for the body to regulate its temperature.

WATER INPUT

WATER OUTPUT

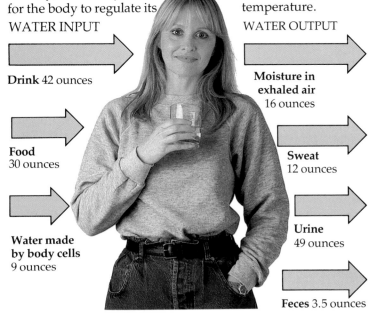

Drink 42 ounces

Food 30 ounces

Water made by body cells 9 ounces

Moisture in exhaled air 16 ounces

Sweat 12 ounces

Urine 49 ounces

Feces 3.5 ounces

HARD OR SOFT WATER – DOES IT MATTER?

Nutritionally, it makes no difference whether you drink hard or soft water, but people on sodium-restricted diets may want to avoid softened water. Water softening removes alkaline minerals like calcium and magnesium, which form hard deposits on utensils, and replaces them with sodium, which leaves no residue.

You take water into your body in liquids and in food. Water is also formed inside the body by the metabolism of carbohydrates, fats, and proteins. The primary ways in which you lose water are in urine (with smaller amounts lost in feces), in sweat, and in moist air breathed out through the lungs.

Tap and mineral water

Both tap and mineral water contain substantial, but highly variable, quantities of minerals. The average person's intake of water, depending on where he or she lives, provides a small percentage of his or her dietary needs for some minerals, such as fluorine, calcium, and magnesium, but a negligible percentage of the dietary needs for most other minerals.

ASK YOUR DOCTOR FIBER AND WATER

Q I have diabetes mellitus and I have been told that a high-fiber diet could help control my blood sugar level. Is this true?

A Yes. Fiber can reduce the high glucose levels found in the blood soon after you eat refined carbohydrates. The bulk of high-fiber foods slows the rate at which sucrose is broken down in your intestines and at which glucose is absorbed.

Q Is a diet that contains a lot of fiber any good for overweight people like me?

A A high-fiber diet could help you lose weight, but not if you simply add fiber to your current diet. The key is to replace high-fat, high-protein foods with those high in complex carbohydrates (starch and fiber). High-fiber foods are low in fat and are more filling than refined foods, so you should feel more satisfied after consuming fewer calories. Along with your change in eating habits, exercising regularly is an essential part of any weight-loss program.

Q I know it's a good idea to drink eight glasses of water a day. But is it possible to drink too much water?

A It is very difficult to drink so much water that the body becomes overloaded. One reason is that your body regulates the absorption of water from the intestine and any excess is excreted in the feces. Increased water intake is compensated for by increased output of urine. In rare instances, people drink excessive amounts of water for psychological reasons. This practice can override some of the body's mechanisms for maintaining water balance.

FOOD TECHNOLOGY

METHODS OF FOOD PRODUCTION, processing, and preservation have developed rapidly over the last hundred years. In general, technology has been beneficial, allowing Americans to choose from an enormous selection of foods from around the world. However, technology brings with it food that is increasingly modified at every stage of its production. This factor has generated questions about exactly what we are eating besides the food itself.

Progress in food processing
Before food processing techniques, people ate only foods recognized as plant or animal or products of agriculture, such as meats, fruits, and vegetables. Technological advances have led to an expansion in the foods available to us. Some examples are shown below.

Rapid advances in food technology have brought a large selection of reasonably priced foods within the reach of an ever-increasing number of people. Processing techniques such as drying, canning, freezing, pickling, and irradiation can increase the shelf life of a vast number of foods. In addition, chemical advances have enabled the creation of completely new types of foods.

Intact food
A food recognized as plant or animal or a product of agriculture is called an intact food.

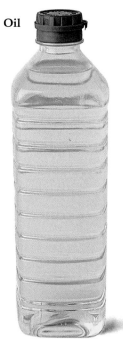

Oil

Grapefruit

Flour

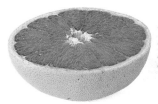

Refined food
A refined food is an intact or partitioned food whose main component is processed to eliminate contaminants and to prolong shelf life. Refined foods are usually used as ingredients.

Margarine

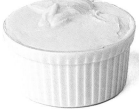

Fabricated food
A fabricated food is made from partitioned foods. It simulates an intact food – being similar to the original in taste, appearance, and texture.

Partitioned food
Using chemical techniques, intact foods can be separated into their constituents, such as fiber, protein, oil, and starch. These are called partitioned foods.

PROCESSING TECHNIQUES

Food-processing techniques prevent the contamination and deterioration of tons of nutritious foods every year. All methods of food preservation act by inhibiting both bacterial activity and the action of natural self-digesting enzymes that break down cells and lead to rotting. They also make food safer by preventing the growth of microorganisms that are dangerous to humans, such as salmonella, *Listeria*, clostridia, *Mycobacterium tuberculosis*, and certain fungi. Natural toxins in food are also destroyed.

Drying
Bacteria and self-digesting enzymes cannot function without water, making drying an important method of food preservation. In the past, foods such as figs, grapes, and dates were laid out in the sun to dry, while foods such as meat and fish were dried by smoking.

Today's high-speed methods allow a wider range of foods to be dried, including milk, eggs, coffee, cocoa, cereal powders, and cereal flakes. These processes keep flavors remarkably close to fresh when the foods are reconstituted.

Freezing
Freezing deprives bacteria and enzymes of water and slows down any chemical reaction that might occur. It does not necessarily kill bacteria or enzymes, but,

so long as the low temperatures are maintained, no bacterial or enzymatic action can occur. Frozen food can be kept for months and even years unchanged. Refrigeration can only slow down (but not arrest) the multiplication of organisms and the action of enzymes.

Heating

Heating to beyond a certain temperature and time destroys bacteria and inactivates enzymes. All common disease-causing bacteria in milk, for example, are eliminated, and other microorganisms are partially eliminated, by pasteurization, in which the milk is heated to 161°F (72°C) for 15 seconds. Thoroughly cooked food contains virtually no dangerous organisms and, if immediately sealed in a vacuum, will keep indefinitely so long as no new bacterial contamination occurs. Alternatively, food can be sterilized by heating it after sealing.

AGRICULTURAL CHEMICALS

Human intervention starts well before the manufacturing process begins. Today, fields are covered with fertilizers and sprayed with herbicides, pesticides, and fungicides. These substances not only ensure healthy crops – they must be used if enough food is to be grown to feed our population economically and without depleting the soil.

The level of concern surrounding the use of chemicals can be measured by scares such as that over a chemical used on apples. The Food and Drug Administration reports that, at the levels approved for use on foods, the chemicals in current use have not been shown to be hazardous to health.

Organic foods

Although all foods, because they are derived from plants or animals, are organic, the term has come to represent foods grown without chemicals and either not

HOW MILK IS PROCESSED

Source
Cows are milked twice a day and the milk is collected daily.

Transportation
The milk is transported in insulated tankers.

Testing
After arriving at the dairy, the milk is tested in the laboratory.

Pasteurization and homogenization
The milk is filtered and pumped over a series of plates, which heat the milk to 161°F (72°C) for 15 seconds, followed by immediate cooling to below 50°F (10°C). Homogenization is a mechanical emulsification process that breaks down the fat into fine particles and disperses the fat throughout the milk so that it will not separate.

Fortification and packaging
The milk is fortified with vitamins A and D and packaged for delivery.

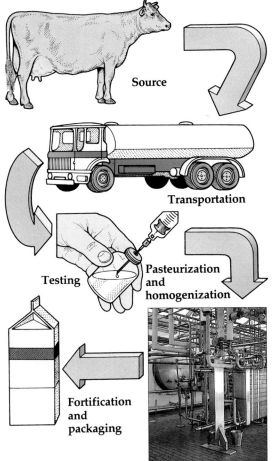

Source

Transportation

Testing

Pasteurization and homogenization

Fortification and packaging

processed or processed without the use of additives. The yield of foods grown without chemicals is relatively low, which makes them expensive, and there is generally more waste from spoilage.

Spraying
Spraying grapevines by helicopter in mid-July ensures that the crop will produce the maximum yield.

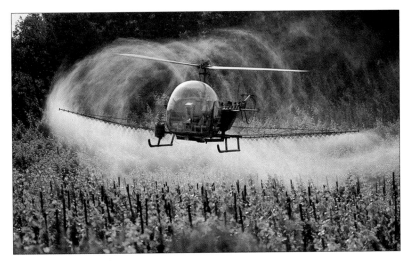

IRRADIATION

Irradiation, in which food is exposed to a radioactive source, destroys bacteria and other contaminants. It does not make food radioactive. Nevertheless, the process has aroused concern. Many people are worried that it may be used to sell substandard food. There is also concern that some vitamins may be destroyed by irradiating food.

As an alternative to other preserving methods, food irradiation is considered reasonable. Controlled irradiation of food reduces the need for pesticides and other chemical methods used in food processing. It can also greatly reduce the need for food additives.

Chemical reactions

Irradiation breaks down long molecules, such as the polysaccharides of cellulose, into smaller carbohydrate molecules. Plant cell walls, which are mainly cellulose, may be affected, causing some fruit and vegetables to soften and bruise.

Irradiation of fat molecules releases free radicals (very chemically active molecular fragments) that oxidize fats and can turn them rancid. Some vitamins, including A, C, and E and the B-complex vitamins, are sensitive to irradiation; the losses are about the same as those that occur in cooking.

FOOD ADDITIVES

Food additives are used to prevent food from spoiling. They also enhance or preserve the natural color and flavor of foods. Additives are rigorously tested for short- and long-term toxicity, and for the effect on human reproduction over at least two generations. The potential ability of an additive to cause mutations in bacteria and cancerous changes is also tested. The amount of additive used is such that the maximum daily intake is much smaller than the amount known through testing to be safe in humans.

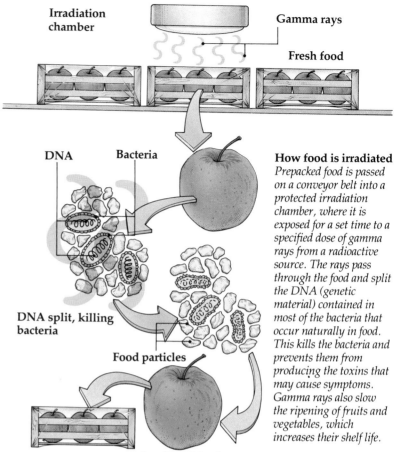

Irradiation chamber · **Gamma rays** · **Fresh food** · **DNA** · **Bacteria** · **DNA split, killing bacteria** · **Food particles** · **Irradiated food**

How food is irradiated
Prepacked food is passed on a conveyor belt into a protected irradiation chamber, where it is exposed for a set time to a specified dose of gamma rays from a radioactive source. The rays pass through the food and split the DNA (genetic material) contained in most of the bacteria that occur naturally in food. This kills the bacteria and prevents them from producing the toxins that may cause symptoms. Gamma rays also slow the ripening of fruits and vegetables, which increases their shelf life.

Additives and cancer

Some research suggests that, on the basis of studies of populations, their diets, and the diseases they suffer, as many as 35 percent of all cancers may be associated with diet. However, although a variety of substances in food have been associated with a higher rate of cancer (see DIET AND CANCER on page 128), very few have definitely been proven to be carcinogenic. In other words, the substances in food that may cause cancer – or possibly prevent it – remain, as yet, largely unidentified.

Much concern has been focused on chemical additives that may be present in food. The estimate that 35 percent of cancers are linked to food is based on studies of people eating natural, unprocessed foods (and possibly contaminants such as fungi). Any contribution to cancer from additives is thought to be extremely small.

IRRADIATION: IS IT SAFE?

Irradiated food is not radioactive. The United Nations Joint Expert Committee on Food Irradiation confirmed in 1970, and again in 1980, that the process was safe. Research has shown that irradiation has little effect on flavor or appearance. The doses needed to kill bacteria without affecting the food are well established. Irradiation can, however, damage the nutritional value by causing the loss of some vitamins sensitive to radiation.

WHAT'S IN YOUR FOOD?

Manufactured foods often contain food additives, which, by law, must be listed on the package. Most packaged foods must also give a complete list of the other ingredients. As an example, the ingredients of a cheesecake mix are listed in the box at right and the additives contained in the mixture, their purposes, and safety are discussed below.

THE INGREDIENTS IN A CHEESECAKE MIX
This cheesecake was made from a mix containing the ingredients listed below plus the additives shown surrounding the picture.

Filling: Sugar, cheese (skim milk, lactic acid, culture); hydrogenated palm kernel, soybean, and coconut oils; corn syrup solids; modified tapioca starch; sodium caseinate (from milk); salt; whey (from milk).

Crust: Enriched flour; sugar; vegetable oil (contains one or more partially hydrogenated oils: coconut, cottonseed, palm, peanut, soybean); eggs; butter; whey (from milk); salt.

THE ADDITIVES IN A CHEESECAKE MIX

FLAVORINGS
In the cheesecake: *Natural flavor; artificial flavor*

Thousands of different flavorings are added to food, usually in very small quantities. Some are essential oils or essences derived from natural sources; others are synthetic copies that are chemically identical to natural flavoring substances. However, the largest group comprises synthetic flavorings developed in the laboratory. They are concentrated and more stable at high temperatures and have a reduced moisture content, making them preferred by many food manufacturers.

THICKENERS
In the cheesecake: *Sodium phosphates*

Most thickeners are obtained from plants. These thickeners include seaweed and algae derivatives and substances produced from cellulose. Examples are agar, guar gum, methylcellulose, and pectin. Large amounts of some thickeners may cause flatulence and abdominal distension.

EMULSIFIERS
In the cheesecake: *Disodium phosphate; propylene glycol monostearate; dipotassium phosphate; monoglycerides and diglycerides; acetylated diglycerides; hydroxylated lecithin*

Emulsifiers are necessary to prevent the oil and water components of many processed foods from separating. As an example, when an egg is used to make mayonnaise or to bind a sauce, the lecithin in the egg works as an emulsifier. For economic reasons, lecithin is now usually produced from soybeans. Other emulsifiers include acacia and polysorbate. There have been reports of some people experiencing allergic reactions to acacia.

PRESERVATIVES
In the cheesecake: *Citric acid*

Preservatives stop or prevent the growth of microorganisms that can cause food poisoning. Because preservatives provide the consumer with safe food at a point distant from the place of production, they are considered safer than food contaminated by bacteria or mold. Common preservatives include nitrates and sulfites. When protein is consumed with nitrates, nitrates may be transformed by bacteria in the intestines into substances called nitrosamines, which are suspected of causing cancer. Sulfites may cause respiratory problems in people who have asthma.

COLORINGS
In the cheesecake: *Artificial color (including yellow 5 and yellow 6)*

Most colors are used for cosmetic reasons. About half are natural pigments such as chlorophyll and beta carotene. Artificial colorings, such as tartrazine, erythrosine, and amaranth, are also widely used. Erythrosine has been shown to affect the thyroid glands of laboratory animals. The link between colorings and hyperactivity in children has never been substantiated in controlled studies. Tartrazine has been implicated in certain allergic reactions.

ANTIOXIDANTS
In the cheesecake: *Butylated hydroxyanisole (BHA)*

Oils and fats in food can become rancid as they slowly combine with atmospheric oxygen. This process, called oxidation, is prevented or delayed by the use of antioxidants. Some antioxidants are natural substances, such as vitamins C and E. Others are synthetic, such as butylated hydroxyanisole (BHA) and butylated hydroxytoluene (BHT). No harmful effects have been found to occur from use of these substances. In fact, limited data suggest they may protect against some forms of cancer.

CHAPTER THREE

YOU AND YOUR DIET

YOUR DIET'S NUTRITIONAL value depends on the foods you choose, on the way in which you store and prepare them, and possibly on the way in which you eat them. This chapter has been designed to help you choose a diet that provides all of the nutrients you and your family need to stay healthy.

The opening section, BALANCING YOUR DIET, will help you determine whether you are fulfilling your requirements. Provided you are eating foods from all the major groups, are thoughtful about the nutrient value of the foods you select, and are maintaining your weight, you are most likely getting all the nutrients you need. But it is useful to make sure that your protein intake is complete, that you are eating adequate amounts of dietary fiber, and that your diet contains foods with sufficient amounts of all the essential vitamins and minerals.

The following two sections, PREGNANCY AND LACTATION and INFANT NUTRITION, review two circumstances that require women to pay special attention to their dietary needs. During pregnancy, a woman needs more calories, protein, calcium, iron, and other nutrients. Breast-feeding requires additional energy to cover the caloric value of the milk and for actual production of the milk. Apart from decisions about whether to breast-feed or bottle-feed, other significant considerations include the age at which you introduce your infant to solid foods.

AVOIDING EXCESS examines the way in which you can cut down on components of your diet, such as saturated fats and foods containing "empty" calories, that may not be helping you. The section on EATING BEHAVIOR focuses on the nutritional effects of how often, and when, you eat. If you eat a balanced diet as a series of small meals rather than two or three large ones, the rise and fall in your blood sugar, insulin, and fats is less dramatic. Also, the overall effect on the level of fat in your blood has been shown to be favorable. In fact, researchers report that eating frequent, small meals can be a useful way to control weight by reducing between-meal hunger.

Finally, the section on FOOD STORAGE AND PREPARATION provides advice on how you can store and cook food in a way that will maintain its maximum nutritional value. MYTH AND REALITY examines some commonly held beliefs (many of them handed down through families and many of them misconceptions) about the value or deleterious effects of certain foods.

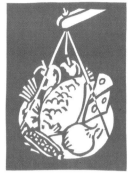

BALANCING YOUR DIET

A BALANCED DIET provides you with food that contains the right mixture of carbohydrates, fats, and proteins, and a sufficient quantity of vitamins and minerals. It also supplies the right amount of calories to fulfill your energy requirements and to maintain your weight. In addition, a balanced diet provides enough fiber and water to allow your digestive system to work efficiently.

There are two primary considerations in balancing your diet. This section reviews the first aspect, which is to ensure that the food you eat contains the proteins, vitamins, minerals, and fiber you need, while at the same time fulfilling your energy requirements. AVOIDING EXCESSES on page 78 discusses a second consideration – how you can avoid taking in too much of any dietary component.

THE MAIN PRINCIPLES

No single food can provide all the nutrients you need. Even using three or four different foods, it would be difficult to create a diet that would satisfy all your nutritional requirements. The best strategy is to eat as many different kinds of naturally occurring foods as possible.

ACHIEVING A BALANCED DIET

The key to healthy eating is a varied diet with the emphasis on ample fluids, high-fiber carbohydrates, a lower intake of fats, adequate protein, and a good mix of naturally occurring foods. Published Japanese dietary guidelines provide one strategy for balancing your diet. These guidelines recommend that you select as many as 30 different kinds of food each day from the groups below. Variety is the key.

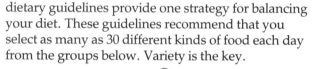

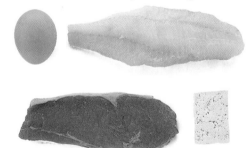

Group 1 Protein sources
Fish, meat, egg whites, soybean products, whole grains, and beans

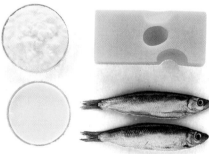

Group 2 Calcium sources
Milk and other dairy products and canned fish with soft bones

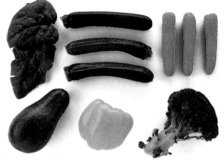

Group 3 Vitamin A sources
Dark green and deep yellow vegetables and orange-yellow fruits

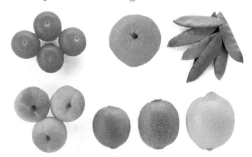

Group 4 Vitamin C and mineral sources
Vegetables and citrus fruits

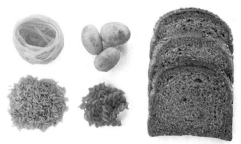

Group 5 Complex carbohydrates
Rice, bread, pasta, and potatoes

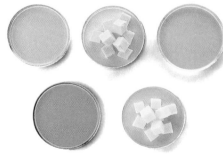

Group 6 Fat sources
Fats and oils

SPECIAL RISK GROUPS

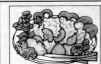

♦ **Infants and growing children** (see INFANT NUTRITION on page 74).

♦ **Vegans, vegetarians, and people whose diets are severely restricted** may find that it requires more attention to achieve a balanced diet.

♦ **Menstruating women**, who may benefit from supplementary iron due to losses of iron in menstrual blood.

♦ **Elderly and solitary individuals** who may have lapsed into an unvarying diet and may need vitamin or mineral supplements.

♦ **People on low-calorie weight-loss diets** and those suffering from anorexia nervosa and bulimia (binge-purge syndrome).

♦ **People who are acutely ill**, such as those who have an infectious disease.

♦ **People who are taking drugs** that interfere with nutrition. For example, if you take certain diuretic drugs, you need more potassium.

♦ **People who abuse alcohol**, especially those who obtain a large percentage of their caloric needs from alcoholic drinks.

♦ **People who have certain chronic diseases** such as diabetes mellitus or kidney disease, or malabsorption syndromes such as celiac sprue.

♦ **Pregnant women**, who need more protein and more of some vitamins and minerals (see PREGNANCY AND LACTATION on page 72).

Fulfilling your nutritional needs is an easy task if you choose the foods you eat wisely. There is little need for complex calculations using tables of the nutritional contents of foods. If you enjoy a well-mixed and varied diet that contains foods from all the major food groups, you are unlikely to suffer any form of nutritional deficiency.

It is important to consider the circumstances that increase your nutritional needs, making special consideration of your diet, and possibly medical advice, necessary. Some of these risk factors are shown in the box above.

ENERGY REQUIREMENTS

The amount of energy provided by food is measured in units called Calories or kilocalories. The amount of energy you need from food depends on how much energy you expend every day. Your daily energy expenditure is made up of two components. First, you expend energy to maintain basic bodily functions, including breathing, heartbeat,

THE CONCEPT OF NUTRIENT DENSITY

"Nutrient density" is a way of evaluating the nutrient richness of a food per number of kilocalories available from that food. For example, a banana and a piece of candy may both provide 100 kilocalories, but the banana also provides some vitamins and minerals; the candy does not. If you eat a lot of food of low nutrient density you will get the calories you need for energy expenditure, but you may fail to get the nutrients you need. A common problem is eating too many "empty-calorie" foods and beverages.

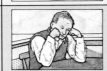

Banana	
CALORIES	100 kilocalories
MINERALS	Phosphorus, calcium, potassium, iron
VITAMINS	Vitamin A, niacin, riboflavin, vitamin B_6

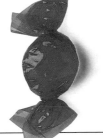

Candy	
CALORIES	100 kilocalories
MINERALS	None
VITAMINS	None

and body temperature. This basal (resting) energy expenditure is about 500 kilocalories a day in a 1-year-old infant, about 1,000 kilocalories a day in an 8-year-old child, and about 1,300 and 1,600 kilocalories a day in an adult woman and man, respectively. There is substantial variation within each group. Energy is also expended in physical activity. The kilocalorie costs per hour of some activities are shown in the chart below. In addition, some energy is required for growth of body tissues. However, even in rapidly growing children, this additional amount is small in comparison with the needs for maintenance (basal) and movement (activity). A pregnant or lactating woman needs at least 300 to 500 kilocalories a day more than her basic needs to provide for the increased demands placed on her body and for the baby's requirements.

Fulfilling your energy requirements

The mechanisms of hunger, appetite, and satiety usually control energy intake and, over time, keep it close to your requirements. In affluent countries, the majority of people have access to an ample food supply and consuming more food than the body needs is a common problem. The people most at risk of insufficient caloric intake are those suffering from poverty, chronic disease, or anorexia nervosa, and people whose appetites have decreased or who may be suffering from physical or mental disabilities that make the preparation and eating of meals difficult.

HOW MUCH ENERGY DO YOU USE?

The number of kilocalories you "burn" during daily activities varies according to your body weight and level of fitness. The amounts given in the chart are for an average fit 154-pound man and an average fit 128-pound woman. The figures do not include the energy required to maintain basal metabolism (see above). They represent only the energy expended during different activities.

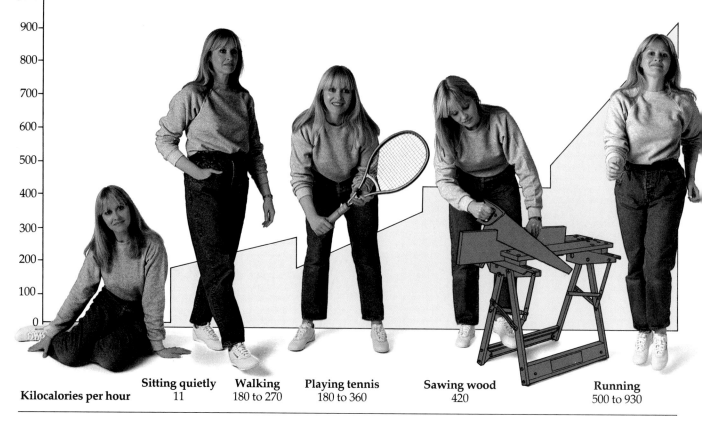

	Sitting quietly	Walking	Playing tennis	Sawing wood	Running
Kilocalories per hour	11	180 to 270	180 to 360	420	500 to 930

WHAT KINDS OF FAT SHOULD YOU EAT?

A substantial proportion of the fat you eat should be unsaturated, with slightly more monounsaturated than polyunsaturated. Butter, lard, and the fats in meats and cheese are high in saturated fat, as are coconut, palm,

and palm kernel oils. Fish oils, most vegetable oils, and some soft margarines are high in unsaturated fat. The relative amounts of the fats in butter and in a variety of vegetable oils are shown below.

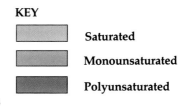

KEY

Saturated

Monounsaturated

Polyunsaturated

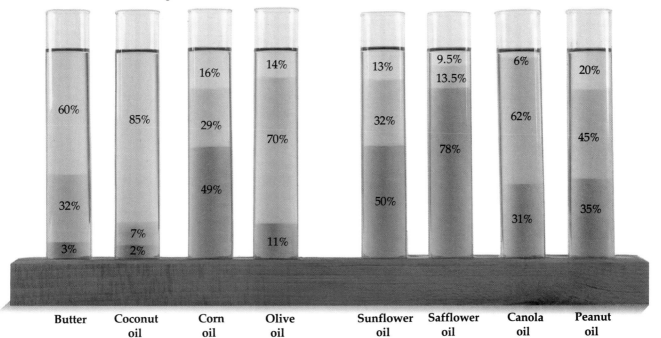

Butter	Coconut oil	Corn oil	Olive oil	Sunflower oil	Safflower oil	Canola oil	Peanut oil
60%	85%	16%	14%	13%	9.5%	6%	20%
32%	7%	29%	70%	32%	13.5%	62%	45%
3%	2%	49%	11%	50%	78%	31%	35%

HOW IS ENERGY MEASURED?

The traditional unit of energy is the calorie, which is the amount of energy needed to heat 1 gram of water by 1° Celsius. For nutritional purposes, calories are impractically small, so the kilocalorie (1,000 calories) is used instead. Kilocalories are sometimes called Calories (with a capital C).

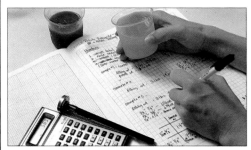

Calculating energy values
To determine a food's energy value, the amounts of carbohydrates, fats, and protein it contains are analyzed. Since the potential energy values of each are known, the energy value is easily calculated.

Sources of energy

Energy comes from two main sources – carbohydrates and fats. About 50 percent of the energy in your diet should be supplied by carbohydrates. Although all types of carbohydrates – sugars and starches – provide similar amounts of energy, sweet-tasting foods usually have more calories in a serving. Nutritionists generally agree that a high percentage of your carbohydrate intake should be eaten in the form of complex carbohydrates. Whole-grain bread, potatoes, rice, whole-wheat pasta, dried peas and beans, fruits, and vegetables are all good complex carbohydrate sources.

Fats are a concentrated energy source. They should constitute no more than 30 percent of your energy needs. The average American obtains closer to 40 percent of his or her calories from fat. The kinds of fats you choose are also important (see box above).

HIGH-FIBER FOODS

Most of the carbohydrates you eat should come from high-fiber foods such as whole-grain bread, whole-wheat pasta, brown rice and legumes, and some fruits. High-fiber foods
♦ are bulkier, making it less easy to overeat
♦ contain minerals and vitamins
♦ make it easy to get the fiber you need.

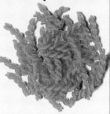

WHAT DIFFERENT PEOPLE NEED

An individual's nutritional requirements vary, partly on the basis of the amount of energy expended and partly on the nutrients needed to grow and support optimum organ and tissue function. You obtain the calories you need for these requirements from the food you eat. The recommended daily calorie requirements and protein needs for different groups of people are given in the boxes. The range of foods that four different people might eat in a week is shown in the photographs.

Carbohydrates should provide about 50 to 55 percent of your energy needs, protein about 15 percent, and fat about 30 percent or less. It has become increasingly apparent that, for those with higher fat intakes, there is every advantage to reducing the amount of fat in the diet. Because people vary greatly in both size and energy expenditure, the figures given here are only approximate.

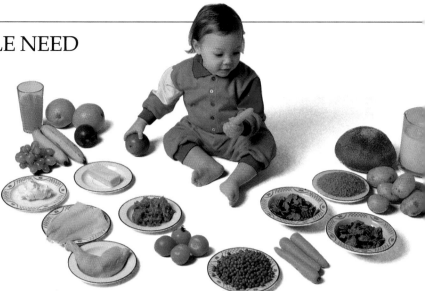

THE RECOMMENDED DAILY INTAKE FOR YOUNG CHILDREN

A child age 1 to 3 needs about 1,000 to 1,300 kilocalories daily. A child age 4 to 6 needs about 1,300 to 1,700 kilocalories a day. Protein needs are determined by body weight – 0.55 grams per pound for a child age 1 to 6.

Young child
The dietary needs of a child of 12 to 24 months are high because the child's metabolic rate is increased by rapid growth and because children of this age are highly active. Serve young children the same foods as everyone else, but in smaller amounts. Don't restrict fat and cholesterol too much and don't overdo high-fiber foods. Sugar and sodium are acceptable in moderation. Young children need the equivalent of 2 cups of milk each day. To get enough calories to grow, many children need higher-calorie foods, such as whole milk.

THE RECOMMENDED DAILY INTAKE FOR TEENAGE GIRLS

An average 16-year-old girl needs about 1,200 to 3,000 kilocalories a day, more if she is an active sports participant. An intake of about 0.41 grams of protein a day per pound ideal weight is recommended.

Teenager
Nutritional needs are particularly high during the rapid physical development that follows puberty. Girls begin to grow earlier and have a peak requirement between the ages of 15 and 18; in boys the peak occurs between 19 and 24 years. All teenagers need three servings of milk, cheese, or yogurt each day to meet calcium needs. If weight is a problem, encourage increased activity rather than dieting.

THE RECOMMENDED DAILY INTAKE FOR SEDENTARY WOMEN

A sedentary, nonpregnant woman age 19 to 34 needs about 1,600 kilocalories a day. Her dietary requirements are different than those of the teenager, but getting enough calcium remains an important element in both diets.

Adult woman
For adult women, food intake and energy expenditure require more attention with each passing decade. The hormonal changes of pregnancy and the hormones ingested from contraceptives encourage the accumulation of fat in the breasts, buttocks, and thighs. The best way to thwart extra weight is by increasing your activity level. A brisk, 2-mile walk taken 5 days a week will help keep you trim.

THE RECOMMENDED DAILY INTAKE FOR ACTIVE MEN

Under conditions of extreme, sustained activity, a very fit man may consume as many as 4,200 kilocalories a day. An intake of about 0.40 grams of protein per pound ideal weight is recommended.

Construction worker
This construction worker requires extra calories to meet his exceptional energy needs and may need slightly more protein to meet the higher-than-average turnover of protein in his muscles. He also needs to eat food with a high carbohydrate content for ready availability of fuel.

COULD YOU LIVE ON MILK ALONE?

No single food can provide all the nutrients you need. The closest single "complete" food is milk, but even milk is not a complete food for a lifetime. It is an inadequate source of iron and is relatively deficient in vitamin C and, unless fortified, vitamin D. Infants are born with a supply of iron that lasts for the first 4 to 6 months. After this time, iron must be supplied by solid foods. Adults can survive without milk since all the nutrients it contains are available in other foods.

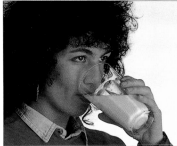

What's in a glass of milk?
Milk is a good source of protein and calcium. Unlike other foods of animal origin, milk contains a significant amount of carbohydrates. Whole milk is high in fat. Low-fat or skim milk may be preferred by people who drink a lot of milk and wish to reduce their fat intake.

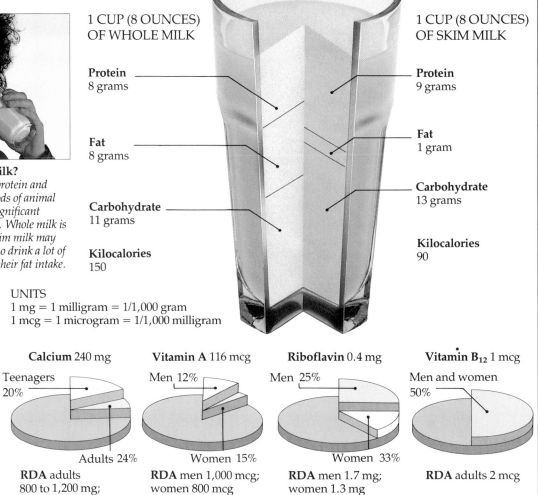

1 CUP (8 OUNCES) OF WHOLE MILK

Protein
8 grams

Fat
8 grams

Carbohydrate
11 grams

Kilocalories
150

1 CUP (8 OUNCES) OF SKIM MILK

Protein
9 grams

Fat
1 gram

Carbohydrate
13 grams

Kilocalories
90

UNITS
1 mg = 1 milligram = 1/1,000 gram
1 mcg = 1 microgram = 1/1,000 milligram

Vitamins and minerals in whole milk
The diagrams show the percentage of the RDAs of some important vitamins and minerals contained in 8 ounces of whole milk. Low-fat and nonfat milk contain similar amounts of calcium, riboflavin, and vitamin B$_{12}$. Milk is fortified with vitamin A by the manufacturer.

Calcium 240 mg
Teenagers 20%
Adults 24%
RDA adults 800 to 1,200 mg; teenagers 1,200 mg

Vitamin A 116 mcg
Men 12%
Women 15%
RDA men 1,000 mcg; women 800 mcg

Riboflavin 0.4 mg
Men 25%
Women 33%
RDA men 1.7 mg; women 1.3 mg

Vitamin B$_{12}$ 1 mcg
Men and women 50%
RDA adults 2 mcg

COULD WE LIVE WITHOUT FAT?

Removing fat from your diet completely is unthinkable. Your body needs a small amount of fat to provide essential fatty acids. A diet that contained no fat would be likely to lead to deficiencies of fat-soluble vitamins.

PROTEIN REQUIREMENTS

Your body uses protein primarily for the maintenance of organs and tissues rather than as an energy source (carbohydrates and fats are more efficient fuel sources). However, if the foods eaten do not provide sufficient energy from carbohydrates and fats, the body will use protein for energy at the expense of the growth or repair needs of cells.

Protein should represent about 15 percent of your total energy consumption. The amount of protein you need every day is determined by your weight and age (see box on RDAS FOR PROTEIN, above right). These recommendations provide considerably more protein than is required to satisfy the needs for basic growth, repair, and maintenance. Most people can fully satisfy their protein needs with two thirds of the recommended daily amount.

RDAs FOR PROTEIN

The figures below show the RDAs for protein, in grams per pound ideal body weight, at different ages. Pregnant women need 10 extra grams of protein daily.

Age (years)	Protein (grams/ pound)
0 to 6 months	1.0
6 months to 1	0.76
1 to 6	0.55
7 to 14	0.45
15 to 18	0.41
19+	0.40

Fulfilling your protein requirements

It is prudent to obtain your protein from several different food sources each day because a variety of sources provides a better mix of micronutrients. The box on page 66 shows the amounts of a variety of foods, each of which contains about 10 grams of protein.

The ability of the body to use different protein sources varies with the characteristics of the source and the proportions of the essential amino acids contained in the proteins. The essential amino acids, which must be supplied in the diet, are methionine, lysine, tryptophan, phenylalanine, isoleucine,

MEETING YOUR FIBER REQUIREMENTS

You should strive for a dietary fiber intake of between 20 and 30 grams a day by eating a variety of different high-fiber foods. Here we show a possible combination of foods that would provide you with a good daily fiber intake.

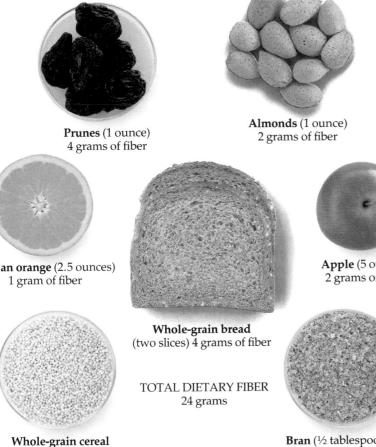

Prunes (1 ounce)
4 grams of fiber

Almonds (1 ounce)
2 grams of fiber

an orange (2.5 ounces)
1 gram of fiber

Whole-grain bread
(two slices) 4 grams of fiber

Apple (5 ounces)
2 grams of fiber

TOTAL DIETARY FIBER
24 grams

Whole-grain cereal
1⅓ ounce) 8 grams of fiber

Bran (½ tablespoon)
3 grams of fiber

ASK YOUR DOCTOR
BALANCING YOUR DIET

Q To be healthy, should my diet provide the recommended daily allowance of all essential nutrients each and every day?

A No. Although our storage capacity for most nutrients (except fat) is limited, the healthy body contains enough reserves of most nutrients to last for many weeks or months. Thus, while recommended intakes are most conveniently expressed in daily terms, it is the overall quality and diversity of the foods you eat over the long term – weeks rather than days – that is most important.

Q Are there some foods that are unquestionably "good" and some that are definitely "bad"?

A The relative value of a food depends on the circumstances under which it is eaten. Pure sugar can be most helpful to a marathon runner but could result in wide swings in the blood sugar of a diabetic. Likewise, an occasional hot dog is not "bad," even though the fat content is high and the nutrient value of this food is modest.

Q I never seem to get enough done in a day. Will taking vitamins give me more energy?

A Vitamins themselves do not have any energy value. They are, however, necessary for the body to use energy that comes from carbohydrates and fats. The B-complex vitamins and the mineral iron are important nutrients for utilizing energy sources. But the best way to get vitamins and minerals is by eating a varied and well-balanced diet.

leucine, threonine, and valine. In general, proteins of animal origin, such as beef, fish, poultry, egg whites, and milk, are high in essential amino acids (and are therefore called complete proteins). Those of vegetable origin, such as peas, beans, nuts, and grains, contain fewer amino acids (and are called partially complete proteins). The white of an egg provides almost perfectly complete protein; close behind it is milk.

No single vegetable protein contains all the essential amino acids. It is possible, however, to get all the essential amino acids by eating a diet of mixed vegetable proteins. For example, grains such as wheat contain about 10 percent protein, are relatively deficient in lysine, but have adequate methionine. Legumes, such as peas and beans, have 20 percent protein, are short of methionine but have adequate lysine. So a mixture of two parts wheat to one part legume has a high biological food value. Peanut butter on whole-wheat bread, or red beans and rice, are also good examples.

VITAMIN AND MINERAL REQUIREMENTS

The section on VITAMINS AND MINERALS on page 36 describes the functions of all the vitamins and minerals that must be supplied by the diet and the common foods in which they are found. By eating a highly varied diet, including plenty of fresh fruits and vegetables, you are likely to obtain all the vitamins and minerals you need. The tables on pages 67 and 70 list some of the circumstances or groups in which the risk of deficiency is increased. These groups include menstruating, pregnant, and lactating women, people on weight-loss diets, some strict vegetarians or vegans, people who have certain illnesses, and people who are taking medications that interfere with mineral or vitamin absorption or that increase the loss of minerals from the body.

GETTING YOUR PROTEIN

Each of the foods below, in the amounts shown, contains approximately 10 grams of protein. It is ideal to eat smaller quantities of a variety of protein-rich foods, rather than a large quantity of just one food. If you choose partially complete protein foods only, select combinations (such as legumes and wheat or rice) that will, in relatively large amounts, provide you with a proportion of the essential amino acids equal to meat or milk.

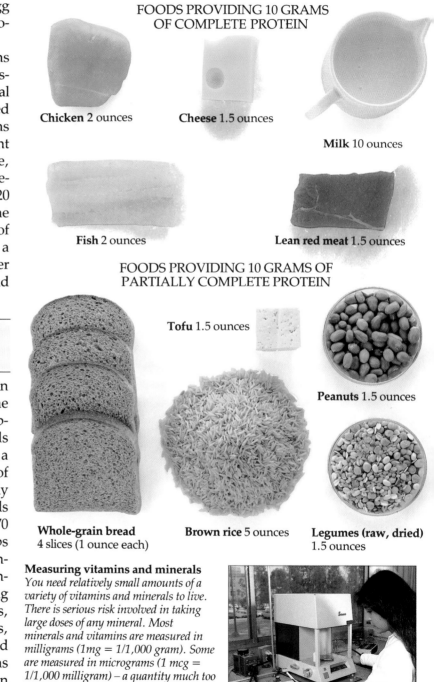

FOODS PROVIDING 10 GRAMS OF COMPLETE PROTEIN

Chicken 2 ounces
Cheese 1.5 ounces
Milk 10 ounces
Fish 2 ounces
Lean red meat 1.5 ounces

FOODS PROVIDING 10 GRAMS OF PARTIALLY COMPLETE PROTEIN

Tofu 1.5 ounces
Peanuts 1.5 ounces
Whole-grain bread 4 slices (1 ounce each)
Brown rice 5 ounces
Legumes (raw, dried) 1.5 ounces

Measuring vitamins and minerals
You need relatively small amounts of a variety of vitamins and minerals to live. There is serious risk involved in taking large doses of any mineral. Most minerals and vitamins are measured in milligrams (1mg = 1/1,000 gram). Some are measured in micrograms (1 mcg = 1/1,000 milligram) – a quantity much too small to be seen by the naked eye.

ARE YOU GETTING ENOUGH VITAMINS?

VITAMIN	RDA (adults)	CIRCUMSTANCES IN WHICH DEFICIENCY MAY OCCUR	DRUGS AFFECTING ABSORPTION
VITAMIN A	0.8 to 1 mg	Deficiency is unlikely if you include orange-yellow or green vegetables, fish, fortified milk, or orange-yellow fruits in your diet. Absorption of vitamin A requires normal digestion of fats; anything that interferes with fat digestion will lead to reduced absorption of vitamin A.	
THIAMINE	1.1 to 1.5 mg	Because thiamine is needed to release energy from carbohydrates, requirements are related to the amount of carbohydrates in the diet. Needs may increase with aging, during periods of increased physical activity, during a feverish illness, and during pregnancy and breast-feeding.	
RIBOFLAVIN	1.3 to 1.7 mg	Deficiency is likely in people on highly restrictive diets and in the elderly. You need more if you are pregnant or breast-feeding and in some cases if you are taking a contraceptive pill. Pregnant women and newborn babies are more liable to suffer riboflavin deficiency than others.	Chlorpromazine (antipsychotic) Amitriptyline (antidepressant)
NIACIN	15 to 19 mg	Deficiency is rare unless the diet is low in protein or the major source of protein is corn. You need more niacin if you are pregnant or breast-feeding.	
PANTOTHENIC ACID	No RDA; suggested intake 4 to 7 mg	Because pantothenic acid is found in a wide variety of foods, deficiency is virtually unknown. However, your needs for pantothenic acid may increase during periods of prolonged stress.	
VITAMIN B$_6$	1.6 to 2 mg	Deficiency is unlikely with any reasonably balanced diet, although intakes may be only marginally adequate unless whole-grain products and chicken or fish are consumed regularly. Women taking contraceptive pills may require a supplement.	Drugs used to treat parkinsonism or epilepsy
VITAMIN B$_{12}$	2 mcg	Deficiency is unlikely if the diet includes foods of animal origin. You are likely to have a deficiency if you are a true vegan or if a portion of your stomach has been removed. Your needs are greater if you drink a lot of alcohol. There are special needs during pregnancy and breast-feeding.	Antibiotics
BIOTIN	No RDA; suggested intake 30 to 200 mcg	Deficiency has occurred in people being fed intravenously. A large intake of raw egg may lead to biotin deficiency, because the vitamin becomes chemically bound to a substance in egg white. Your needs increase if you are taking a contraceptive pill or drink a lot of alcohol.	
FOLIC ACID	180 to 200 mcg	Deficiency is unlikely with any well-balanced diet. Needs increase during pregnancy and breast-feeding and during prolonged infection, certain types of anemia, bowel disease, cancer, and leukemia. You may also need more if you are taking a contraceptive pill or drink a lot of alcohol.	Many drugs, including aspirin, antacids, and some anticonvulsants
VITAMIN C	60 mg	Deficiency is unlikely with a diet containing fresh fruit and vegetables. You are more at risk of deficiency if you smoke, drink a lot of alcohol, take a contraceptive pill, are suffering from an infectious disease, or are undergoing dialysis. Needs increase during pregnancy and breast-feeding.	
VITAMIN D	5 to 10 mcg	Long-term regular use of mineral oil or conditions that interfere with fat absorption can reduce the body's uptake of vitamin D. People who are never in the sun could be at risk of deficiency since vitamin D is also formed in the skin by the action of sunlight.	Anticonvulsants Some antibacterials Some sleeping preparations
VITAMIN E	8 to 10 mcg	Deficiency is almost unknown but needs increase during pregnancy.	
VITAMIN K	60 to 80 mcg	Deficiency is unlikely if the diet includes plenty of plant foods but may occur if you have liver disease or a fat malabsorption disorder.	Some anticoagulants Some antibiotics

FOUR NUTRITIOUS MEALS

Each of these meals contains substantial amounts of proteins and carbohydrates, some fat, and a selection of important vitamins and minerals. If you vary the fruits and vegetables and the sources of proteins and carbohydrates you eat at meals and as snacks throughout the day, you will achieve a balanced diet.

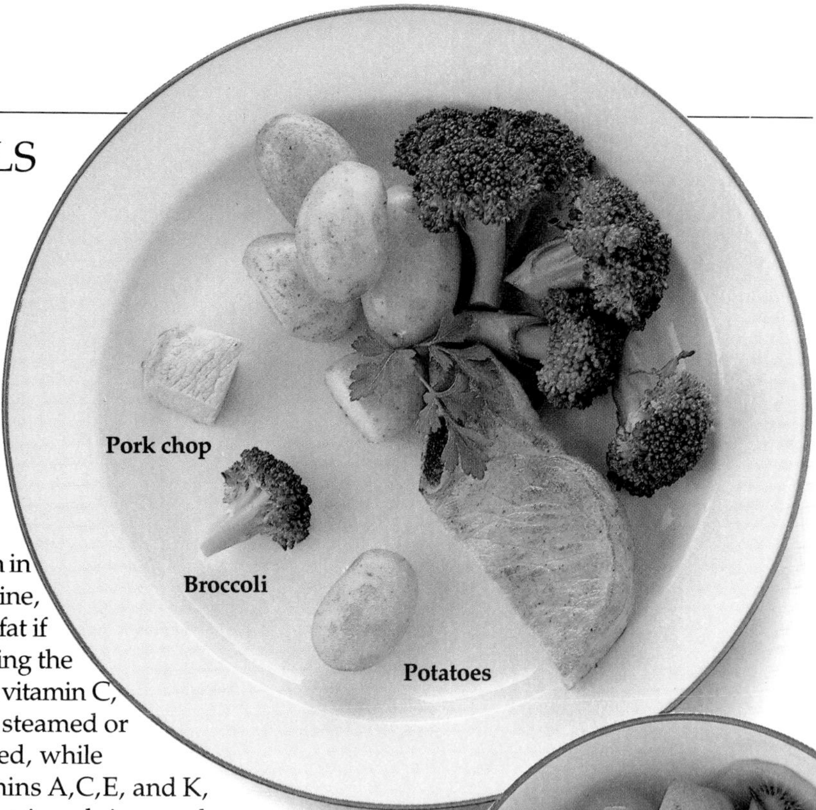

AMERICAN

Broiled pork chop
New potatoes
Broccoli
Fruit salad

Pork is an excellent source of protein, is rich in phosphorus and thiamine, and is relatively low in fat if it is broiled after trimming the fat. Potatoes are rich in vitamin C, particularly if they are steamed or baked rather than boiled, while broccoli contains vitamins A,C,E, and K, folic acid, and the minerals iron and calcium. The fruit salad is particularly high in vitamin C.

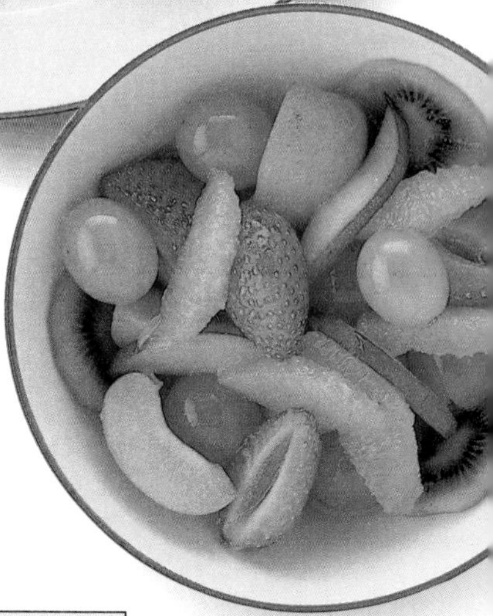

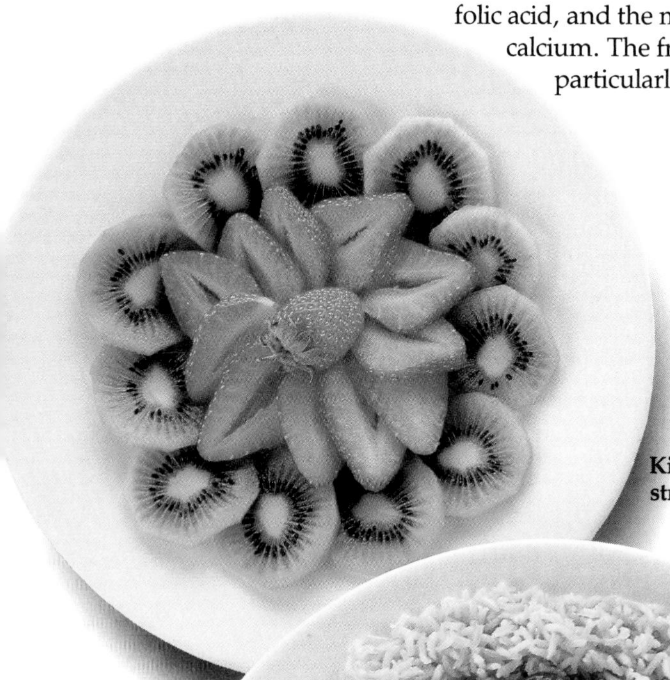

Pork chop

Broccoli

Potatoes

Fruit salad

Kiwi fruit and strawberry salad

VEGETARIAN

Chili-baked beans
Brown rice
Green salad
Kiwi fruit and strawberry salad

This bean dish is rich in both protein and fiber, while also being a good source of B vitamins and minerals. The amino acids in the rice complement those in the beans, providing a complete protein. The rice is also an excellent source of energy, B vitamins, and magnesium. The green salad and fruit dessert score well for vitamin C.

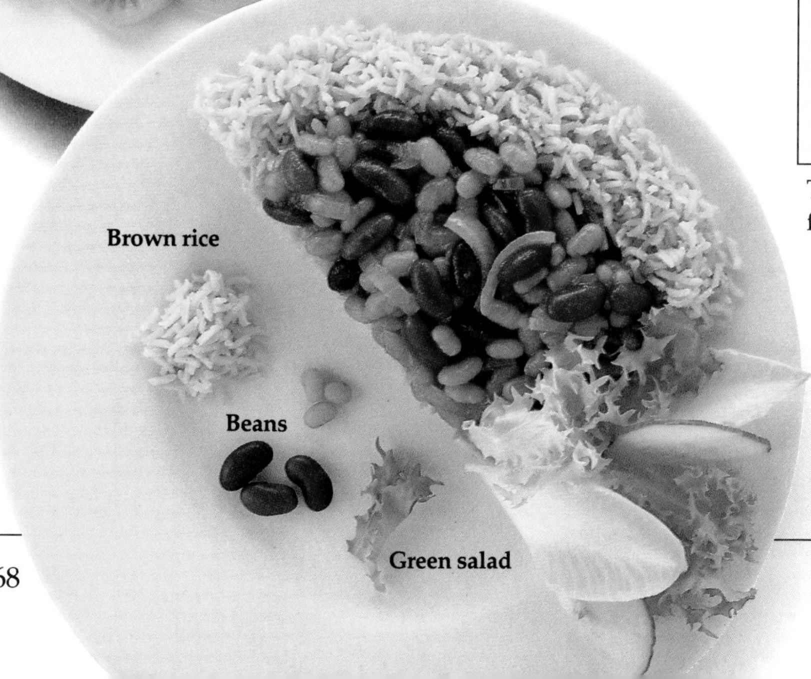

Brown rice

Beans

Green salad

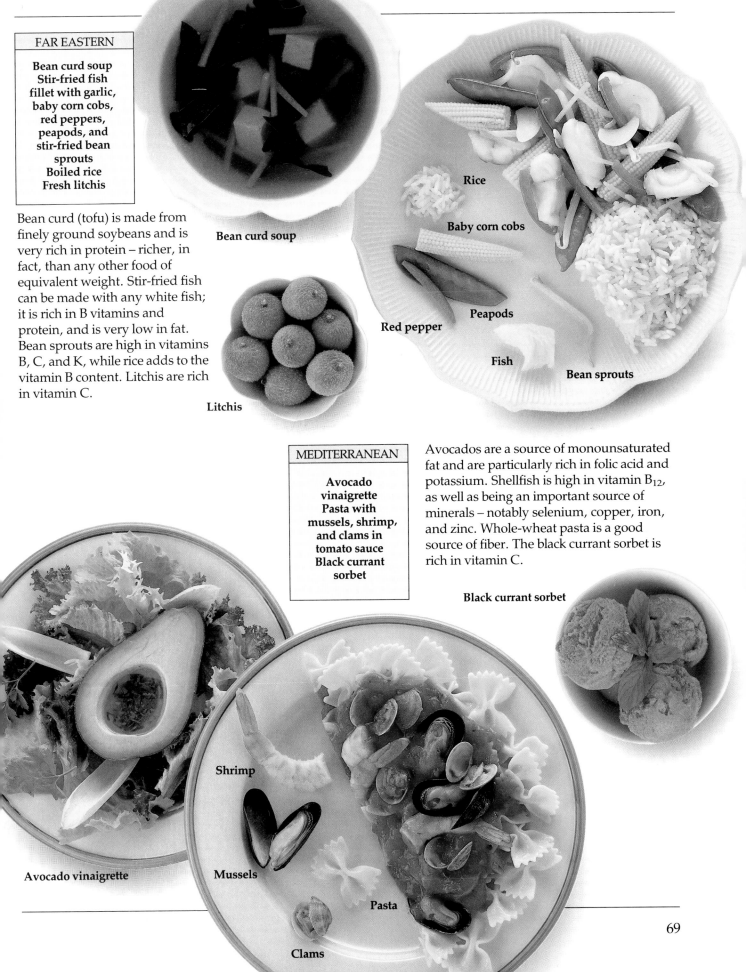

FAR EASTERN

**Bean curd soup
Stir-fried fish
fillet with garlic,
baby corn cobs,
red peppers,
peapods, and
stir-fried bean
sprouts
Boiled rice
Fresh litchis**

Bean curd (tofu) is made from finely ground soybeans and is very rich in protein – richer, in fact, than any other food of equivalent weight. Stir-fried fish can be made with any white fish; it is rich in B vitamins and protein, and is very low in fat. Bean sprouts are high in vitamins B, C, and K, while rice adds to the vitamin B content. Litchis are rich in vitamin C.

Bean curd soup

Litchis

Rice

Baby corn cobs

Peapods

Red pepper

Fish

Bean sprouts

MEDITERRANEAN

**Avocado
vinaigrette
Pasta with
mussels, shrimp,
and clams in
tomato sauce
Black currant
sorbet**

Avocados are a source of monounsaturated fat and are particularly rich in folic acid and potassium. Shellfish is high in vitamin B_{12}, as well as being an important source of minerals – notably selenium, copper, iron, and zinc. Whole-wheat pasta is a good source of fiber. The black currant sorbet is rich in vitamin C.

Black currant sorbet

Avocado vinaigrette

Shrimp

Mussels

Pasta

Clams

ARE YOU GETTING ENOUGH MINERALS?

MINERAL	RDA (adults)	CIRCUMSTANCES IN WHICH DEFICIENCY MAY OCCUR	DRUGS AFFECTING ABSORPTION
CALCIUM	800 to 1,200 mg	Deficiency can occur if the diet contains insufficient quantities of calcium-rich foods such as milk, cheese, yogurt, and greens. Poor digestion and absorption of fats in the intestine may reduce absorption of calcium. A diet that is too high in fiber can also reduce absorption.	Neomycin Tetracycline
IODINE	150 mcg	Deficiency has occurred in isolated areas fed by glacial water supplies and where the only food available is grown in iodine-poor soil. Anyone who lives in such an area and does not use iodized salt could be at risk of deficiency and goiter.	
IRON	Men 10 mg; women 15 mg	Iron is needed for synthesis of hemoglobin. It is relatively easy to become deficient, especially if you have heavy or frequent menstruation or donate blood regularly. For this reason, women often require iron supplements. The best source of iron is red meat. Needs increase during pregnancy.	
MAGNESIUM	Men 350 mg; women 280 mg	Deficiency can result from excessive losses through severe diarrhea, alcohol abuse, and prolonged use of certain types of diuretics.	
POTASSIUM	No RDA; suggested intake 3.5 g	Deficiency rarely occurs from insufficient dietary intake but can result from severe diarrhea or vomiting, or from kidney disease. A high intake of sodium (salt) causes loss of potassium.	Insulin Diuretics Adrenocortical steroids
SELENIUM	Men 70 mcg; women 55 mcg	Deficiency is unlikely to occur except in people eating foods from restricted geographical areas where there are low levels of selenium in the soil.	Diuretics
ZINC	Men 15 mg; women 12 mg	Deficiency may occur in children and in the elderly. It may also occur with a rare congenital defect of zinc absorption or when a special synthetic medical diet (oral or intravenous), which is zinc-free, is given. Pregnant and lactating women have increased needs.	Diuretics Penicillamine (antirheumatic)

Are vitamin and mineral supplements necessary?

Supplements may be beneficial for people whose risk of deficiency is increased. The question of whether vitamin or mineral supplements are of demonstrable use to anyone else is more controversial. While full-blown vitamin- or mineral-deficiency diseases are uncommon today in the US, some health professionals believe that marginal deficiencies are widespread. Proponents of vitamin supplements argue that modern food processing reduces the nutrient content of food. Today's stressful life-style may also increase the tendency to faulty eating practices as well as the need for certain nutrients, particularly vitamins C and E and vitamin B complex.

The long-term solution to these problems is to improve your diet and re-examine your life-style. Extend the range of foods you eat, including fresh fruit, vegetables, whole-grain cereals, and nuts. In addition, try to eat foods in as fresh a state as possible and without excessive cooking. Finally, cut down on foods that are low in micronutrients but high in calories, such as ice cream, cakes, soda, and alcoholic drinks.

Bear in mind that supplements are not a substitute for basic food elements.

Types of supplements
Shown here are examples of supplements that may be needed in special circumstances. Ask your doctor before taking any supplement.

Vitamin B₁₂

Iron

Folic acid

CASE HISTORY
A POORLY BALANCED DIET

Ruby MADE AN APPOINTMENT **with her doctor because she was troubled by persistent bad breath, which she found both unpleasant and embarrassing. She had not seen her dentist in several years, and wanted to see her doctor anyway because she had several other concerns. Most of them she considered minor and probably insignificant, but they had been bothering her.**

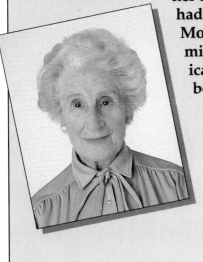

PERSONAL DETAILS
Name Ruby Littleton
Age 69
Occupation Homemaker
Family Ruby was widowed 12 years ago, when she was left with very little money. She has no family and few friends and hardly ever leaves her apartment.

MEDICAL BACKGROUND
For a person who has exercised little throughout her life, Ruby's health has been remarkably good. Although she has an occasional migraine headache, what really concerns her is constant fatigue. She has never been in a hospital and has not seen her doctor for several years.

THE CONSULTATION
Ruby tells her doctor about her bad breath. He checks her gums and sees that they are swollen, red, spongy, and bulge out between her teeth. Ruby tells him that she has pain when she brushes her teeth and her gums bleed. Further examination reveals extensive bruising on her left thigh and shins and, on most parts of her body, pinpoints of bleeding around the roots of the hairs. The doctor examines her skin and finds that the hairs are deformed and spiral-shaped.

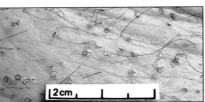

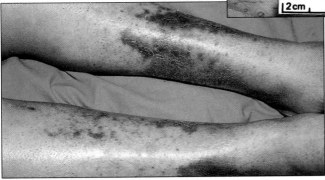

Symptoms of scurvy
In people suffering from scurvy, hairs on most parts of the body become corkscrew-shaped (above) and bruising also occurs very easily, as seen here on the shins (left).

FURTHER INVESTIGATION
Ruby's doctor takes a blood sample, which shows that she is anemic. His suspicions aroused, he asks her about her diet. Ruby tells him that, because she has been too tired to shop, she has been living entirely on cheese, crackers, canned sardines, cookies, and black coffee for more than a year.

Another blood sample taken in the hospital reveals a very low level of vitamin C in Ruby's blood platelets, confirming her doctor's suspicions about the cause of her illness.

THE DIAGNOSIS
Ruby is suffering from a variety of problems, the most serious of which is SCURVY, a severe deficiency of vitamin C. None of the foods she has been eating contain this vitamin.

THE TREATMENT
Along with a balanced diet, Ruby is prescribed 250 milligrams of vitamin C four times a day, which is enough to saturate her body. The doctor explains to her that vitamin C is essential to the health of the cells between the capillaries of her gums. Without it, the capillaries ooze. In addition, the bacteria that usually live harmlessly in her mouth have attacked her damaged gums, causing infection. Within a month, the condition of Ruby's gums has improved, her mouth infection has cleared up, and her bruises, also caused by weak capillaries, have disappeared.

THE FOLLOW-UP
Ruby reads several books on nutrition. She now eats a well-balanced diet, with plenty of orange juice, fresh fruit and vegetables, protein, and fat. She also has the energy to take a walk every day and to shop for her fruit and vegetables at the corner fruit stand.

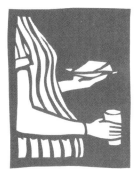

PREGNANCY AND LACTATION

CAREFUL ATTENTION to your nutritional requirements is important during pregnancy and lactation, both for your own sake and for that of your baby. It has also become increasingly apparent that, to give your baby the best possible start in life, it is wise to eat well even before you conceive.

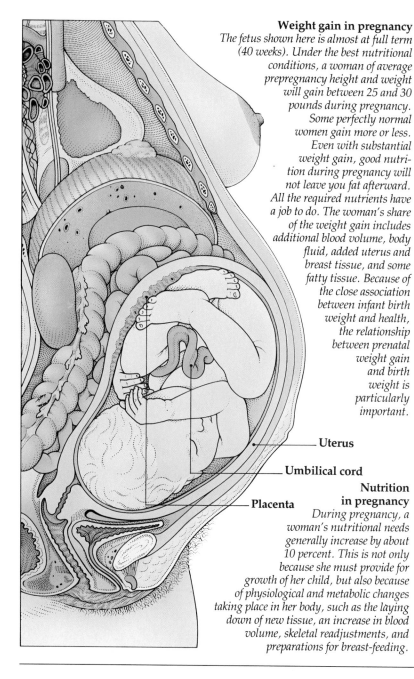

Weight gain in pregnancy
The fetus shown here is almost at full term (40 weeks). Under the best nutritional conditions, a woman of average prepregnancy height and weight will gain between 25 and 30 pounds during pregnancy. Some perfectly normal women gain more or less. Even with substantial weight gain, good nutrition during pregnancy will not leave you fat afterward. All the required nutrients have a job to do. The woman's share of the weight gain includes additional blood volume, body fluid, added uterus and breast tissue, and some fatty tissue. Because of the close association between infant birth weight and health, the relationship between prenatal weight gain and birth weight is particularly important.

Uterus

Umbilical cord

Nutrition in pregnancy
Placenta
During pregnancy, a woman's nutritional needs generally increase by about 10 percent. This is not only because she must provide for growth of her child, but also because of physiological and metabolic changes taking place in her body, such as the laying down of new tissue, an increase in blood volume, skeletal readjustments, and preparations for breast-feeding.

Your requirements for energy, protein, vitamins, and minerals increase during pregnancy and lactation. For most women, these increased needs can be achieved through a well-balanced diet. For maximum benefit to mother and baby, good dietary habits should be established well before conception.

BEFORE CONCEPTION

Significant changes in the fetus occur at a very early stage in pregnancy, and the environment in which the fetus develops and grows is influenced by the state of your body before your pregnancy starts. If you have a metabolic disorder such as diabetes mellitus you should ask your doctor for help in controlling the condition before conception.

Dietary preparation for pregnancy also includes stabilizing your weight.

ALCOHOL AND SMOKING

Most physicians recommend that you eliminate alcohol and smoking during pregnancy.

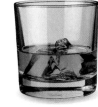

In general, women who smoke more than 15 cigarettes a day have infants who weigh 150 to 200 grams less than infants born to women who smoke less, or who do not smoke.

LACTATION

You need an additional 500 kilocalories a day if you are breast-feeding. Requirements for vitamins A, E, and C, thiamine, riboflavin, niacin, zinc, and iodine increase. Your need for protein, vitamin B$_6$, and folic acid decreases in comparison to pregnancy.

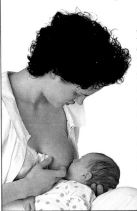

Nutrition during lactation
The quantity of breast milk is maintained by the stimulus of regular nursing, but the quality of the milk is influenced by the mother's diet. It is important to make sure that you eat properly.

Another concern is the stores of vitamins in your body. Research studies have shown that an adequate intake of folic acid is particularly important if you have already had a baby with a neural tube defect (spina bifida or a related disorder). Many doctors recommend a supplement for a few months before conception and during the first trimester.

CALORIE AND PROTEIN INTAKE

Healthy women are advised to increase their calorie intake by about 300 kilocalories a day after the first month of pregnancy. Throughout pregnancy, you should eat an additional 10 to 15 grams of protein a day beyond the daily requirement of about 45 grams. You can take care of both your increased need for calories and protein by adding 3 cups of skim milk to your daily diet. For variation, use cottage cheese, yogurt, and fish, chicken, and lean red meat.

The extra calories and protein are needed for growth of the fetus and placenta, as well as for growth in the size of the uterus and in the amount of supporting tissue, including breast tissue.

VITAMINS AND MINERALS IN PREGNANCY

Along with increased calorie and protein requirements during pregnancy there are increased needs for vitamins and minerals. In most cases, these needs are met as a result of increased food intake. If you have doubts about the quality and quantity of your diet, your doctor may recommend supplements. Although supplements are valuable, they do not take the place of a well-balanced diet and are intended only as extras.

CALCIUM

Calcium is better absorbed during pregnancy than at other times and there is little likelihood of your becoming deficient during pregnancy and breast-feeding if you eat and drink plenty of calcium-rich foods. You need about 1,200 milligrams of calcium a day. Your selection should include at least 32 fluid ounces of milk.

Cheese 1 ounce
200 milligrams of calcium

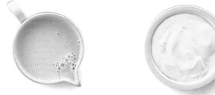

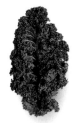

Milk 32 ounces
720 milligrams of calcium

Yogurt (plain) 8 ounces
400 milligrams of calcium

Kale 4 ounces
250 milligrams of calcium

IRON

You need about 30 milligrams of iron per day during pregnancy. Iron is found mainly in red meat and liver and other organ meats. Iron supplements are often prescribed during the second and third trimesters and for 2 to 3 months after delivery to ensure that your body stores are replenished. This is particularly important for vegetarians and vegans.

Kidney beans 3 ounces
5 milligrams of iron

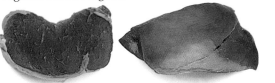

Red meat 8 ounces
6 milligrams of iron

Calf liver 6 ounces
18 milligrams of iron

Chicken liver 6 ounces
12 milligrams of iron

ZINC

The levels of zinc in the blood usually fall by about 30 percent during pregnancy. There are some suggestions that a zinc intake below half the recommended daily amount of about 20 milligrams is associated with a poor intake of protein and, thus, smaller-than-average babies.

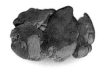

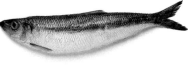

Herring 1 ounce
30 milligrams of zinc

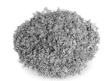

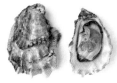

Wheat germ 1 ounce
4 milligrams of zinc

Oysters 1 oyster
22 milligrams of zinc

Walnuts 3 ounces
2.8 milligrams of zinc

INFANT NUTRITION

A BABY GROWS MORE RAPIDLY during the first year than at any other time in his or her life. In fact, by the age of 6 months, a baby usually has doubled his or her birth weight. A good diet, containing the right amounts of carbohydrates, fats, proteins, vitamins, and minerals, is essential for your baby's health and is also important in establishing healthy eating patterns.

During the first three to six months, most babies' nutritional requirements can be met by either breast milk or formula. Breast-feeding has both psychological and nutritional advantages over bottle-feeding. Human milk provides the perfect balance of nutrients. It also contains antibodies that protect the baby against infection. However, so long as commercially manufactured formulas are prepared according to the instructions and the baby receives sufficient physical closeness during feedings, bottle-feeding is a satisfactory method.

The breast-fed baby
Let your baby regulate his or her intake of breast milk by nursing as long as the baby wants. Breast milk at the end of the feeding has more fat and protein than the milk that is produced at the beginning. An infant who is allowed only a limited time to nurse at each breast may not obtain enough milk to satisfy his or her hunger.

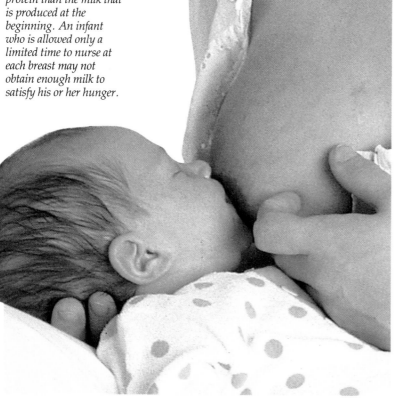

BREAST-FEEDING

The Committee on Nutrition of the American Academy of Pediatrics strongly recommends that healthy, full-term infants be breast-fed for the first few months after birth.

Breast milk – the perfect food
In the first few days after birth, the mother's breasts secrete a special type of milk called colostrum, which provides all the water and other nutrients that most babies need. If a baby is persistently hungry or simply requires more calories than he or she can get from breast-feeding, formula may be offered after the initial feeding. If feedings are offered frequently after milk has come in, no further supplementation is usually needed.

Colostrum contains less fat and more protein, vitamin A, vitamin E, thiamine, sodium, and potassium than mature milk. It also contains antibodies, which help protect the baby against intestinal organisms and allergens.

The composition of breast milk changes to that of mature milk over a period of about 10 days. The constituents of mature breast milk remain the same but the proportions of these constituents vary during every feeding and at different times of the day. The milk at the beginning of the feeding is watery and acts as a thirst quencher; the milk toward the end contains about five times as much fat and one and a half times as much protein.

WHEN NOT TO BREAST-FEED

Many drugs taken by the nursing mother, including prescription drugs and drugs of abuse, are secreted in breast milk. This is also true of alcohol. If you are breast-feeding your baby, your milk has the potential for transmitting these substances to your baby. The safest course is to check with your doctor before taking any drugs, including alcohol.

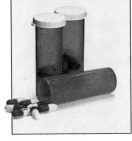

BOTTLE-FEEDING

Commercial formulas are designed to provide the baby with all the necessary nutrients. However, one disadvantage of bottle-feeding is that the person who is giving the bottle may feel that the baby should finish every drop. This can lead to overfeeding.

The best approach is to offer the baby a bottle when he or she seems to be hungry. Try to be "tuned in" to your baby's indications that signal hunger. Also, be aware of the signals that could mean that your baby is not interested in feeding at the moment, such as turning the head from side to side when offered (or while drinking from) a bottle or not sucking. But also keep in mind the frequency with which a baby must be fed. Feeding "on demand" should gradually evolve into a fairly regular schedule.

Premature infants

The nutritional requirements of low-birth-weight and premature infants are higher than those of full-term infants. Special nutritionally enriched formulas have been designed to meet the needs of the low-birth-weight or premature infant. These formulas support growth better than breast milk alone does because they contain the additional vitamins needed by these infants. In other cases, breast milk is obtained from the mother and is supplemented with vitamins before being given to the infant.

Types of bottles
Many shapes and sizes of bottles and nipples are available. Some bottles may be purchased already filled with formula.

COMPOSITION OF DIFFERENT MILKS

The charts compare the average composition of mature human milk with milk-based infant formula and whole cow's milk. Cow's milk is much more concentrated in minerals, particularly sodium and potassium, so it is difficult for the infant's kidneys to process. Cow's milk and other animal milk is also unsuitable for infants because the protein content is too high and the carbohydrate content is too low. Most of the protein in cow's milk is in the form of curds; in human milk the more digestible whey predominates. The whey is also nutritionally superior in its protein composition. Infant formulas modify cow's milk to more closely resemble breast milk. The protein is modified and its content is lowered, and butterfat is replaced by vegetable oils.

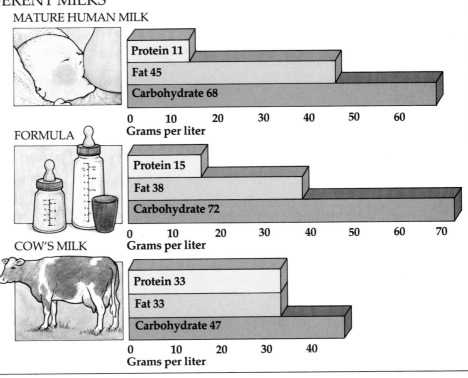

MATURE HUMAN MILK

Protein 11
Fat 45
Carbohydrate 68

0 10 20 30 40 50 60
Grams per liter

FORMULA

Protein 15
Fat 38
Carbohydrate 72

0 10 20 30 40 50 60 70
Grams per liter

COW'S MILK

Protein 33
Fat 33
Carbohydrate 47

0 10 20 30 40
Grams per liter

MONITOR YOUR SYMPTOMS
SLOW WEIGHT GAIN IN BABIES

The weight of babies under 1 should be carefully monitored because failure to gain weight normally may indicate an underlying health problem. Your baby's pediatrician will probably weigh your baby regularly and will tell you if there is any cause for concern. You may also want to keep your own records, which you can compare with the standard figures for normal babies of the same birth weight, as shown on the opposite page. Consult the diagnostic chart below if your baby seems to be gaining weight too slowly.

WEIGHT LOSS DURING THE FIRST WEEK OF LIFE

It is normal for babies to lose up to 5 ounces in the first week after birth. There is no need to worry that your milk supply is inadequate or that your baby is ill. On about the fifth day, babies usually start to gain weight, achieving their birth weight by about the tenth day and gaining weight steadily thereafter.

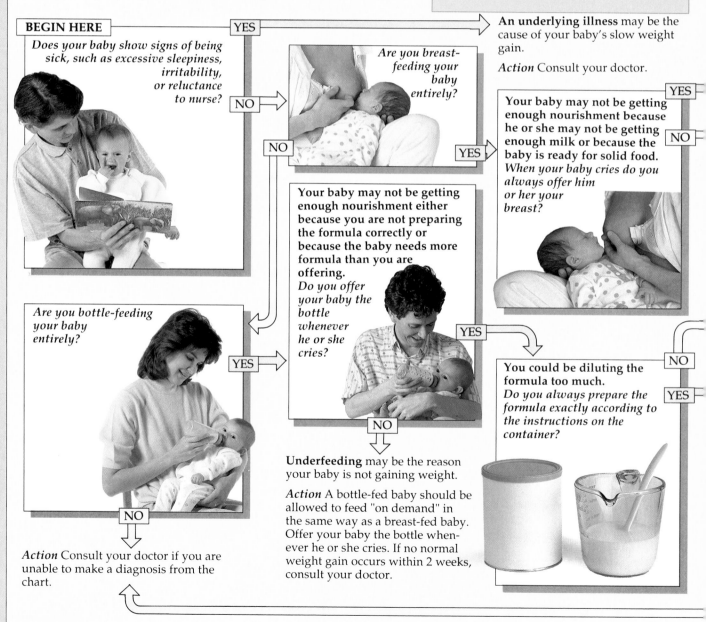

BEGIN HERE

Does your baby show signs of being sick, such as excessive sleepiness, irritability, or reluctance to nurse?

YES

An underlying illness may be the cause of your baby's slow weight gain.

Action Consult your doctor.

NO

Are you breast-feeding your baby entirely?

NO

YES

Your baby may not be getting enough nourishment because he or she may not be getting enough milk or because the baby is ready for solid food. *When your baby cries do you always offer him or her your breast?*

YES

NO

Your baby may not be getting enough nourishment either because you are not preparing the formula correctly or because the baby needs more formula than you are offering.
Do you offer your baby the bottle whenever he or she cries?

Are you bottle-feeding your baby entirely?

YES

YES

NO

You could be diluting the formula too much.
Do you always prepare the formula exactly according to the instructions on the container?

NO

YES

Underfeeding may be the reason your baby is not gaining weight.

Action A bottle-fed baby should be allowed to feed "on demand" in the same way as a breast-fed baby. Offer your baby the bottle whenever he or she cries. If no normal weight gain occurs within 2 weeks, consult your doctor.

NO

Action Consult your doctor if you are unable to make a diagnosis from the chart.

RECORDING WEIGHT GAIN

The three solid curves represent standard patterns of growth in head circumference and weight gain for small, average, and large babies. The case plotted here (dots) represents an average-sized baby who is gaining too little weight. The head is growing normally, but weight gain is slowing down.

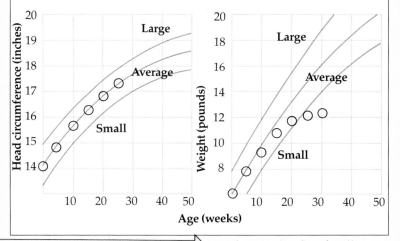

INTRODUCTION TO SOLID FOODS

Doctors recommend that solid foods be introduced at about 4 to 6 months of age, when your infant is able to sit up with support and has good control of his or her head and neck.

At this stage of development, your baby will be able to indicate a desire for food by opening his or her mouth and leaning forward, and to indicate lack of interest by leaning back and turning his or her head away. Remember, however, that the age at which solid foods are introduced cannot be set rigidly. The timing depends largely on your baby's growth rate, stage of development, and level of activity. Your baby's pediatrician can help you make a decision on when to offer solid foods.

On the basis of current knowledge, there is no medical or nutritional advantage to introducing solid foods before 4 to 6 months of age.

What foods should your baby eat?

At the age of 4 to 6 months your infant's ability to masticate with the gums and swallow solid foods is more developed; in addition, the digestive system is mature enough to allow digestion. Introduce single-ingredient foods of soft, moist texture one at a time every few days. The sequence of foods is not critical, but iron-fortified, single-grain infant cereals are a good early choice. Later, the addition of individual (not mixed) vegetables, fruits, meats, and dairy products such as yogurt and cheese, will introduce your child to a variety of foods and set the pattern for a diversified diet in later life.

During the nursing period, infants require little supplemental water. However, once you begin to introduce solid foods, it is a good idea to offer water from a cup or a bottle. Continue breast-feeding or bottle-feeding your infant, but remember that cow's milk is too concentrated in protein and minerals for your infant's kidneys.

Underfeeding may be causing your baby's slow weight gain.

Action Always give your baby the chance to nurse whenever he or she cries. If you stick to a rigid feeding timetable you may be depriving your baby of a sufficient amount of milk and you may also be diminishing your milk supply. If, after you have been nursing on demand for 2 weeks, your baby still is not gaining weight, consult your doctor.

Inadequate intake of milk may be the problem. Other causes include an inadequate maternal diet, or illness, fatigue, drug use, or smoking by the mother. If your baby is more than 3 months old, he or she may be ready for weaning.

Action It is important for the mother to be healthy and to know when to discontinue breast-feeding, so consult your doctor. You may be advised to give supplementary bottles or to start the baby on solid food.

Incorrect mixing of the formula may mean that your baby is receiving insufficient nourishment.

Action Always make sure you use the correct proportion of water to powder or liquid concentrate.

Some babies grow faster and have more rapidly increasing appetites than others. Your baby may need more food than he or she is being offered, even though it is the recommended amount for his or her age.
Does your baby always finish the bottle completely?

YES

NO

Your baby's increasing nutritional requirements may mean that he or she needs more food than you are giving.

Action Always offer your baby more milk and allow him or her to drink until satisfied.

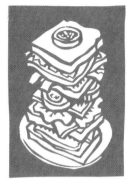

AVOIDING EXCESS

THE PRINCIPAL DIETARY PROBLEM for many sedentary people living in developed countries is that food consumption exceeds what is necessary to fulfill the body's energy requirements. If, in addition, the diet is unbalanced and contains too much fat, cholesterol, and refined (low-fiber) carbohydrate, overeating can intensify any genetic predisposition a person may have for disorders ranging from obesity to maturity-onset diabetes.

So prevalent is the pattern of excessive eating among the increasingly sedentary populations of developed countries that the health of nearly everyone would benefit from increased activity and a reduced intake of food.

THE CONSEQUENCES OF OVEREATING

Many people eat so much food that they receive more than enough protein, carbohydrates, and fats. However, if the foods they eat are high in fats and sugar, and do not include whole grains, green leafy vegetables, and fruits, these people may not receive sufficient amounts of vitamins, minerals, and trace elements.

Body fat
Any calorie intake that exceeds energy and body maintenance requirements is deposited under the skin and within the abdomen as fat. The unneeded dietary fats, carbohydrates, and protein are converted into a fat that may stimulate production of new fat cells and/or expand any existing fat cells.

Obesity
Reducing your intake of fat is the most important step in preventing obesity. Fats provide, weight for weight, more than twice the calories of carbohydrates or proteins. Yet we often eat too much fat because eating high-fat foods is a pleasant and fast way of taking in the

NUTRITION WITHOUT EXCESS

Breakfast **Mid-morning snack**

tbsp = tablespoon
tsp = teaspoon

Lunch

The foods pictured here would supply the 1,600 kilocalories of energy needed by a 5 foot 11 inch, 170-pound woman, age 45, whose work is not physically demanding and whose leisure activities do not include prolonged physical exertion. The day's menu illustrates that a higher-fat, fast-food lunch can be balanced with lower-fat items at breakfast and dinner.

	Shredded wheat 2 biscuits	Low-fat (2%) milk 1 cup	Orange juice ¾ cup	Apple 4 ounces	Burger 2 ounces, in bun	French fries 2 ounces	Catsup 1 tbsp	Cola drink 8 fluid ounces
ENERGY, in kilocalories	178 kcal	145 kcal	90 kcal	61 kcal	243 kcal	137 kcal	16 kcal	96 kcal
PROTEIN, in grams	5 g	10.3 g	1.2 g	0.2 g	18.8 g	2.2 g	0.3 g	. . .
FAT, in grams	1 g	4.9 g	0.6 g	0.6 g	8.6 g	6.6 g	0.1 g	. . .
CARBOHYDRATE, in grams	40 g	14.8 g	21 g	15.3 g	21.2 g	18 g	3.8 g	37.2 g
DIETARY FIBER, in grams	5.5 g	. . .	. . .	2 g	2 g	1 g	. . .	. . .

calories we need for energy and body maintenance. Remember that your body's caloric requirements are quickly met and exceeded by fats. For this reason, it is useful to choose high-fiber, low-energy carbohydrates as your main energy source. These types of foods help abolish your hunger pangs without providing as many calories.

Diabetes and other diseases

The tendency to have diabetes, a disorder in which the pancreas produces insufficient amounts of or no insulin, runs in some families. Non-insulin-dependent (maturity-onset) diabetes develops gradually and mostly in people over 40. A high proportion of the people genetically predisposed to this disease go on to acquire it. Significantly, the people in whom diabetes develops are primarily those who are overweight.

Obesity has also been associated in population studies with coronary heart disease, gout, arthritis, and disorders of the reproductive cycle. All these disorders are common in an overnourished population. Gallstones, for example, are strongly associated with obesity and diets that are high in fat.

HOW OBESITY CAN CAUSE ABNORMAL GLUCOSE TOLERANCE

Insulin mediates the passage of glucose from the blood into body cells. In a trim person the pancreas produces as much insulin as the cells require. In overweight people, usually those over 40, insulin may be sufficient only to ensure cell function with smaller reserves for periods of stress.

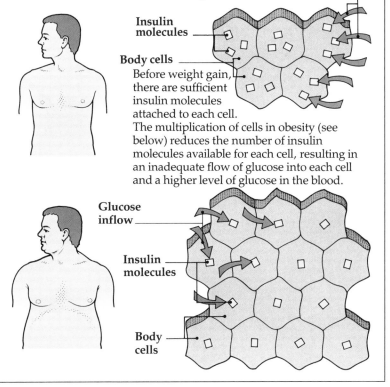

Before weight gain, there are sufficient insulin molecules attached to each cell.

The multiplication of cells in obesity (see below) reduces the number of insulin molecules available for each cell, resulting in an inadequate flow of glucose into each cell and a higher level of glucose in the blood.

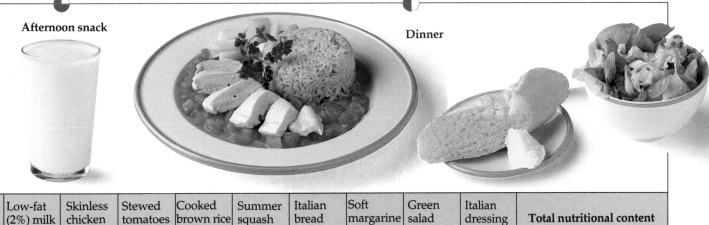

Afternoon snack   **Dinner**

Low-fat (2%) milk 1 cup	Skinless chicken 3 ounces	Stewed tomatoes ½ cup	Cooked brown rice ½ cup	Summer squash ½ cup	Italian bread 1 slice	Soft margarine 1 tsp	Green salad 1½ cups	Italian dressing 1 tbsp	**Total nutritional content**
145 kcal	161 kcal	31 kcal	116 kcal	14 kcal	28 kcal	34 kcal	18 kcal	83 kcal	1,596 kcal
10.3 g	30.6 g	1.5 g	2.4 g	0.9 g	0.9 g	...	1.3 g	...	85.9 g
4.9 g	3.3 g	0.2 g	0.6 g	0.1 g	0.1 g	3.8 g	0.1 g	9 g	44.5 g
14.8 g	...	6.6 g	24.8 g	3.2 g	5.6 g	...	3.3 g	1 g	230.6 g
...	...	1.5 g	3 g	1.5 g	0.5 g	...	0.5 g	...	17.5 g

TOO MUCH FAT

A diet high in fats is a risk to your health because it results in large quantities of low-density lipoproteins, or LDLs (see page 32) in the blood. LDLs increase when you eat fats from foods such as meats, dairy products, and tropical oils (e.g., coconut or palm oil) and in cocoa butter (e.g., chocolate). People who have high levels of LDLs in their blood are at greater risk of heart disease. On the other hand, a diet high in polyunsaturated fats, such as those found in certain vegetable and fish oils, lowers the levels of LDLs and increases the relative proportion of high-density lipoproteins (HDLs) in the blood. This blood composition appears to be associated with lower rates of heart disease.

All fats contain about the same number of calories per serving. Whatever the levels of high-density or low-density lipoproteins, a high intake of fat in sedentary people leads to obesity.

FATS AND ATHEROSCLEROSIS

Atherosclerosis is a degenerative process of the arterial wall in which the inner layer thickens. Too much cholesterol in the blood, resulting from too high an intake of fats or from a genetic tendency to high levels of cholesterol in the blood, forms raised areas on the inner walls of the arteries that can reduce or completely obstruct blood flow.

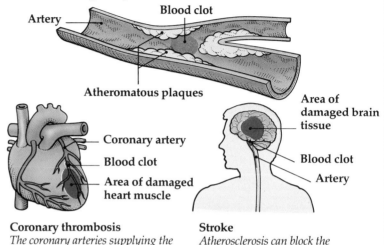

Coronary thrombosis
The coronary arteries supplying the heart with blood can become blocked by atherosclerosis and blood clots, resulting in damage or death to the heart muscle.

Stroke
Atherosclerosis can block the arteries that supply the brain with blood, leading to damage or death of an area of brain tissue.

WHY CHOOSE FRIES?

French fries purchased from a fast-food restaurant can be high in saturated fats. While an occasional meal of this type is not unhealthy, if you are trying to reduce your fat intake, consider some alternatives. A crisp salad with low-fat dressing provides a vitamin-rich accompaniment to your fast-food hamburger. At home, try baked potatoes or whole-grain bread, which contain little or no fat.

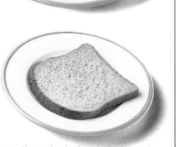

A standard portion of fries contains
Weight: 4 ounces **Energy:** 300 kilocalories **Saturated fat:** 4 grams

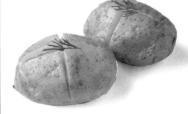

A baked potato contains
Weight: 12 ounces
Energy: 240 kilocalories
Saturated fat: 0.2 grams

One slice of whole-grain bread contains
Weight: 1 ounce
Energy: 67 kilocalories
Saturated fat: 0.1 grams

TOO MUCH REFINED CARBOHYDRATE

To produce refined foods such as white flour, white sugar, or polished white rice, manufacturers first remove a large proportion of fiber from the raw foodstuffs. Because of this, the consumption of refined foods often goes hand-in-hand with a diet that is low in fiber. Eating too much refined carbohydrate tends to contribute to obesity and is usually associated with a high intake of fat. In addition, because of their association with a low-fiber diet, refined carbohydrates are considered to be a causative factor in several bowel disorders.

Constipation is one of the most common problems in developed countries, yet it is rare in populations that are accustomed to eating a high-fiber diet. An increased intake of fluids and dietary fiber rapidly relieves the symptoms of constipation by increasing the bulk and softness of the stools and shortening the transit time through the bowel. An increase in dietary fiber of about 10 grams usually relieves constipation. High-fiber diets are also widely recommended to treat irritable bowel syndrome, diverticular disease, and hemorrhoids.

While high-fiber diets are useful, your diet should not contain too much fiber; 30 grams or more per day can cause gas and bowel irritability. In addition, if your diet is low in animal protein, the absorption of vital minerals can be compromised by a high-fiber diet. If moderate amounts of fiber are eaten, mineral absorption is not adversely affected.

High-fiber carbohydrate foods are important in the management of diabetes because they modulate the body's absorption of glucose during digestion. However, although diet control is essential in the treatment of insulin-dependent diabetes, there is no evidence that nutritional factors play any role in causing this form of the disease.

DENTAL CARIES

Dental plaque is a coating that can develop on and between the teeth. It has a base of sticky, complex sugars that are broken down by bacteria in the mouth. These complex sugars also provide a constant source of nourishment for the bacteria when all other food has been washed away. The process by which the bacteria metabolize the sugars produces acids that cause dental caries (tooth decay). This process is aided by rich sources of sucrose (table sugar), especially if these sugars are in a form that stick to the teeth.

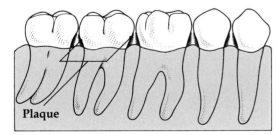

Plaque

1 When not removed by brushing or flossing, deposits of plaque appear in sheltered sites between the teeth.

ADDED FATS AND ADDED SUGAR

Many processed foods contain a surprisingly large amount of saturated fat and refined carbohydrate (the latter usually in the form of added sugar).

High fat
Potato chips and other snack items
Sausages
Luncheon meats

High sugar
Catsup
Bottled sauces
Canned fruit in syrup
Soft drinks
Some breakfast cereals

High fat and sugar
Cookies
Cakes
Pastries
Ice cream
Pies
Cream desserts

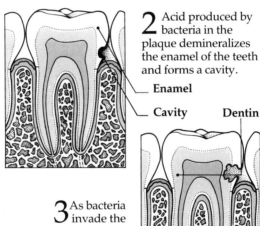

2 Acid produced by bacteria in the plaque demineralizes the enamel of the teeth and forms a cavity.

Enamel

Cavity   **Dentin**

3 As bacteria invade the cavity, it enlarges and the dentin is exposed.

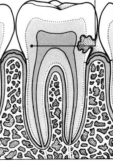

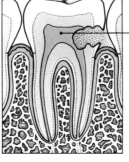

Pulp

4 Finally, the bacteria reach the pulp at the center of the tooth. If the cavity is not cleaned and filled, the infection will eventually destroy the tooth.

BLOOD CHOLESTEROL

For most people the main determinant of blood cholesterol levels is the quantity of saturated fats that is eaten. Eating foods high in cholesterol, such as egg yolks, on a regular basis over time also elevates your blood cholesterol level. However, the main determinant of cholesterol in the blood is your intake of saturated fat. Tropical oils (e.g., palm or coconut oil) and cocoa butter are rich in saturated fat but contain no cholesterol and yet have the effect of raising blood cholesterol levels.

DIVERTICULA AND A LOW-FIBER DIET

Diverticula are small pouches or pockets of the lining of the colon, the main section of the large intestine. The cause of diverticula is uncertain, but they are believed to be associated with too low an intake of fiber. Diverticula are rare in developing countries, where fiber consumption is high. However, in developed countries, they affect more than half the population by age 80. Vegetarians, who have a much higher fiber intake than nonvegetarians, are much less prone to diverticula.

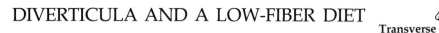

Transverse colon

Where do diverticula occur?

Diverticula are rare in the ascending colon, where the feces have a high liquid content. However, as the fecal material travels through the transverse and descending colon, it begins to solidify. The highest incidence of diverticula occurs in the sigmoid colon. None are found in the rectum.

Ascending colon

Sigmoid colon

Descending colon

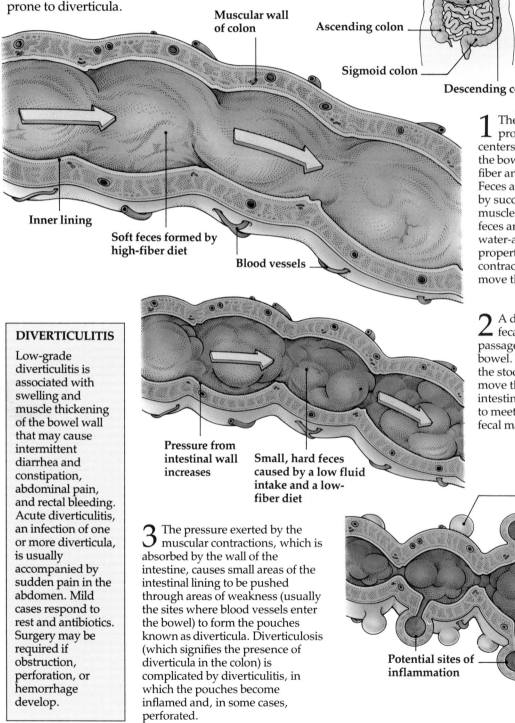

Muscular wall of colon

Inner lining

Soft feces formed by high-fiber diet

Blood vessels

1 The most popular theory proposed to explain diverticula centers on the differences between the bowel contents of people on high-fiber and those on low-fiber diets. Feces are moved through the bowel by successive contractions of the muscles in the bowel walls. If the feces are kept soft and bulky by the water-attracting and water-retaining properties of a high-fiber intake, the contractions of the intestinal muscles move the contents swiftly forward.

2 A diet low in fiber results in less fecal material and in slower passage of fecal material through the bowel. More water is absorbed, and the stools become small and hard. To move the stools, the force of the intestinal contractions increases, only to meet resistance from the hardened fecal material.

DIVERTICULITIS

Low-grade diverticulitis is associated with swelling and muscle thickening of the bowel wall that may cause intermittent diarrhea and constipation, abdominal pain, and rectal bleeding. Acute diverticulitis, an infection of one or more diverticula, is usually accompanied by sudden pain in the abdomen. Mild cases respond to rest and antibiotics. Surgery may be required if obstruction, perforation, or hemorrhage develop.

Pressure from intestinal wall increases

Small, hard feces caused by a low fluid intake and a low-fiber diet

3 The pressure exerted by the muscular contractions, which is absorbed by the wall of the intestine, causes small areas of the intestinal lining to be pushed through areas of weakness (usually the sites where blood vessels enter the bowel) to form the pouches known as diverticula. Diverticulosis (which signifies the presence of diverticula in the colon) is complicated by diverticulitis, in which the pouches become inflamed and, in some cases, perforated.

Diverticula are forced through weaknesses in muscular wall

Potential sites of inflammation

TOO MUCH SALT

As with so many nutritional recommendations, moderation is the key to salt intake. Don't severely restrict your salt intake unless your doctor recommends it. Restriction is usually advised for people who are genetically predisposed to hypertension (high blood pressure) or who have problems with fluid retention.

When there is too much salt in the diet, the body maintains its salt balance by increasing the amount of salt excreted in the urine. Conversely, healthy people on a low-salt diet rarely become depleted of sodium because their kidneys conserve sodium by reducing the excretion in the urine.

As explained in Chapter One, societies with very low average salt intakes have a lower incidence of hypertension. People in developed countries on the average consume more salt than they need.

TOO MANY VITAMINS

For people who eat a balanced diet, the routine use of over-the-counter vitamin supplements carries the risks of vitamin excesses and imbalances. Because the fat-soluble vitamins A, D, and K are stored in the liver and body cells, too much of any of these can have a toxic effect that results in a wide range of health problems, including headache, nausea and vomiting, dizziness, hair loss, abdominal pain, and bone pain. Most of these problems disappear once the excessive use of vitamins has stopped. Children are particularly susceptible to vitamin A and D poisoning. The other fat-soluble vitamin, E, is not known to be toxic. However, vitamin E increases tissue storage of vitamin A, which illustrates the complex relationship among vitamins. Sometimes an excess of one vitamin can raise requirements for others, so it is best to ask your doctor if you think you need a particular vitamin supplement.

CHOOSING FOODS WISELY

Balance is the key to avoiding excess in your diet. Nutritionists recommend selecting the foods in your diet from the widest possible variety of naturally occurring foods. Combine this advice with a program of regular exercise, which will help you use most efficiently the energy from the foods you eat.

TRY TO AVOID

♦ **Excess body weight.** Obesity may place you at a higher risk of hypertension, coronary heart disease, and maturity-onset diabetes. If you are overweight, your calorie intake is exceeding your energy expenditure (see WEIGHT GAIN AND OBESITY on page 98).

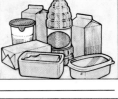

♦ **Too much fat.** In developed countries, about 40 percent of the calories eaten come from fats (saturated and unsaturated). Try to reduce this figure to 30 percent or less in your diet. Fat intake is not considered to be too low unless it falls below 10 percent of your total calorie intake.

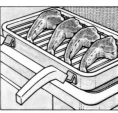

♦ **Saturated fats.** Change to low-fat milk, switch to low-fat cheese, cut out butter, eat margarine high in polyunsaturated fats, cut out solid fats (such as lard), and use vegetable oils such as corn, canola, sunflower, olive, safflower, or soybean oils. Eat lean meat and grill or broil your food rather than fry it.

♦ **Too many refined foods.** Refined foods include polished rice, white flour, and white sugar. They are not the nutritional equivalent of the complex, unrefined forms. Minerals and vitamins are lost by refining and most are not replaced by enrichment.

CHOOSE INSTEAD

♦ **Fiber-rich complex carbohydrates.** Complex carbohydrates are found in whole-grain products, brown rice, peas, dried beans, and fresh fruits and vegetables. These foods are richer in vitamins and minerals than their refined counterparts.

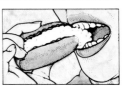

♦ **Carbohydrates as your primary energy source.** Get a larger proportion of your energy from carbohydrates. If carbohydrates now provide 45 percent of your calories, raise the total to 55 percent.

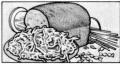

♦ **Foods containing fiber.** Try eating more fiber if your current intake is too low. You don't necessarily need 30 grams of fiber every day. In fact, too much fiber can upset your digestive system or lead to decreased mineral absorption.

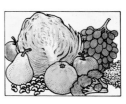

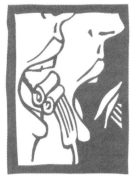

EATING BEHAVIOR

EATING PATTERNS VARY GREATLY among individuals and cultures. Not only do people eat different foods, they take meals with different frequency and place a wide range of values on the social importance of mealtimes. For many Americans, scheduling a family dinner around work commitments, school functions, and recreational activities is a major achievement.

Just as the people of different countries eat different foods, so the manner in which food is perceived as part of tradition and the environment in which it is eaten varies from one culture to another.

THE WAY PEOPLE EAT

In southern Europe, mealtimes are much more than eating times. They are often prolonged social occasions, with the whole family sitting together at the table for several hours at a time. This convivial scene can still be found in the US today, although the social importance of mealtimes seems to be diminishing under the demands of work and leisure activities.

Eating meals in restaurants is an important part of social life here, as it is in other countries. However, most families have neither the income nor the inclination to eat out every night.

In surveys of food shoppers across the country, about one quarter of the people said that the ease and speed of preparation were the most important considerations in making food purchases. More than one third of the people surveyed said they rarely had more than half an hour to prepare meals.

After a hectic day at work, the ideal dinner would be one that is nutritious and appealing, as well as easily and quickly prepared.

EATING PATTERNS

Primitive peoples spent many hours each day searching for fruits, roots, berries, nuts, vegetables, and any small birds or animals that came their way. Anthropologists have found that people ate whenever food was available. Sometimes long periods passed between these

Different ways of eating
A meal can be an important social occasion, with the entire family sitting around the table and talking for several hours. It can be a celebration with a close friend or a solitary occasion consisting of a quick bite at a hamburger stand.

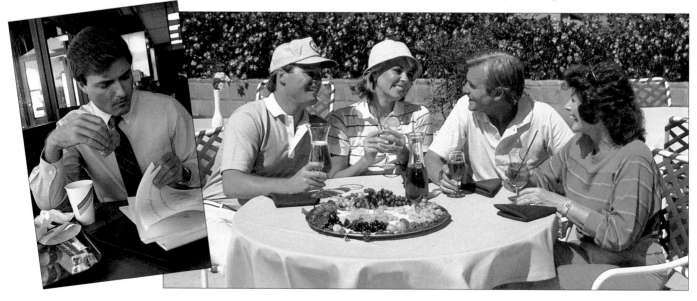

times. Primitive humans mainly sub-sisted on small amounts of low-calorie foods and, on rare occasions, feasted together after a successful hunt.

Some nutritionists believe that our metabolisms evolved over thousands of years of this life-style to deal with a limited food supply. Certainly, the stomach is capable of storage. A meal can be chewed and swallowed in just a few minutes and then digested over a period of several hours.

In this respect, some humans are more like carnivores, such as lions or wolves, than herbivorous animals, such as rabbits, cows, or chimpanzees, which spend the greater part of the day periodically eating a variety of plant foods.

Eating frequent small meals – sometimes called grazing – is considered the best way to control weight since the "grazer" is less likely to feel hungry, as he or she might between large meals.

In fact, a recent US study reported that a group of men who ate frequent small meals throughout the day lowered their blood cholesterol levels compared with a group who ate the same amount of food in three large meals. Based on this evidence, eating small amounts of food frequently may be beneficial – provided the foods have a high nutrient content and do not add up to too many calories.

Conserving energy

Because the food supply was limited in primitive times, we are conditioned to conserve energy. Eating one or two large meals a day may trigger this conservation mechanism. Whenever there is a long interval between eating, it signals to the body that there is an absence of available food. In response, the body becomes more efficient at conserving energy, which can lead to weight problems.

If the same number of calories is consumed throughout the day with short intervals between eating, there is no need for the body to conserve energy because the food supply is continuous.

HEALTHY SNACKS AND DESSERTS

Healthy eating doesn't mean that you can't treat yourself to delicious snacks and desserts.

SNACKS

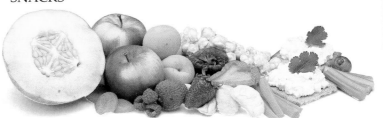

Lightly salted, air-popped popcorn

Fresh seasonal fruits, such as apples, apricots, bananas, cherries, melon, oranges, pears, peaches, pineapple, and plums

Dried fruits, such as apricots, dates, figs, prunes, and raisins

Raw vegetables, such as carrot and celery sticks, slices of zucchini and cucumber, rings of green or red pepper, and cherry tomatoes

Whole-grain crackers spread with cottage cheese or peanut butter

DESSERTS

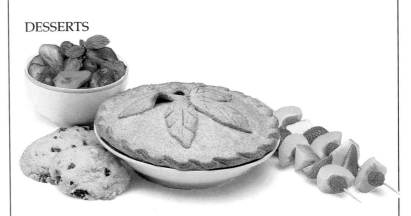

Fresh fruit sundae, made by topping frozen yogurt with unsweetened fresh fruit and nuts

Slice of whole-wheat flour fruit pie, made with a single rather than a double crust to reduce fat and calories

Oatmeal raisin cookies, made using less fat and sugar than your usual recipe

Fruit kabob, made by threading colorful combinations of fresh fruit, alternated with small cubes of cheese, on a skewer.

Fruit compote, made by cooking apples, peaches, or berries, flavored with cinnamon, in a small amount of water, until just tender

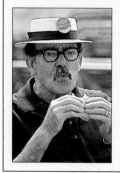

Research studies have documented the fact that more food energy is given off as heat with frequent feedings than if the same amount of food energy is consumed in one or two larger meals. This mechanism is also the reason why fasting does not produce the dramatic weight loss you would expect with such a low food intake.

FAST FOODS

Eating at fast-food restaurants is more popular than ever. Why do we do it? The reasons are clear – quick service, convenience, and a product that is predictable. At a time when Americans are more interested than ever in the nutritional value of their food, it's a good idea to understand what you're getting when you eat a fast-food meal.

Most fast foods provide some of the nutrients you need, including protein and some vitamins and minerals. What they often don't provide are vitamin A, vitamin C, and calcium. Another drawback is the high fat, sodium, and calorie content of fast foods relative to the nutrients they provide. The low fiber content of fast foods is another concern.

Many fast-food establishments are adding salad bars, where you can choose fruits, greens, and other vegetables. Add only small amounts of creamy salads and dressings if you want to keep the nutrient content high and the fat content low.

If a sandwich is your preference, the plain, small hamburgers are a better choice than the deluxe ones, which usually have twice the amount of meat and are often accompanied by high-fat, calorie-rich sauces and cheese.

Fast-food fish and chicken are typically batter-fried and are thus higher in fat and calories than a small hamburger. Delicatessens provide a better variety of healthy eating options. Turkey breast (or other lean meat) on whole-grain bread accompanied by a garden salad is an excellent choice.

ONE CHOICE

Pancakes and maple syrup
High in both fat and sugar if made with whole milk and eggs

Hot dog with mustard and catsup, french fries, and a milk shake
Low in vitamins and high in fat, salt, and sugar

Cola and potato chips
High in sugar, fat, and salt

Sweet-and-sour pork and spring roll
High in fat, sugar, and salt

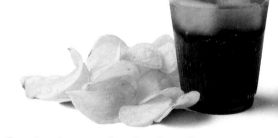

A BETTER CHOICE

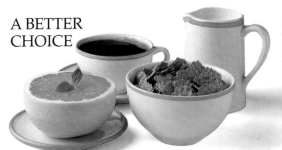

Bran flakes, low-fat milk, grapefruit, coffee
Low in fat and high in fiber, minerals, B-complex vitamins, and vitamin C

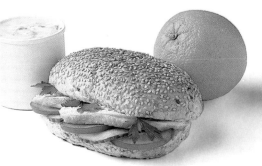

Chicken sandwich, fruit, yogurt
High in vitamins, minerals, and fiber and low in fat

Apple, air-popped popcorn, orange juice
High in vitamins, minerals, and fiber and low in fat and sugar

Vegetable soup, stir-fried beef and vegetables
High in vitamins, minerals, and fiber and low in fat

Convenience foods have also moved beyond their earlier, high-fat, high-salt image. Many quickly prepared, healthy options are now available. Look for chicken, fish, or lean-meat entrées that are broiled or roasted. Check the labels for the salt and fat content. It is not difficult to choose wisely if you follow the guidelines you use for fresh food.

Time-saver cooking

"What shall we have for dinner?" If you, like many people, echo this refrain (especially Mondays through Fridays), consider the following methods of preparing and serving nutritious meals.

Perhaps most important is having an adequate supply of food in the house. Keep your cabinets, freezer, and refrigerator stocked with fresh foods and packaged ingredients, such as rice and beans, that can be used in a variety of ways.

There is no need to spend a lot of time on every component of the meal. If your main dish requires preparation time, carrot sticks and a simple salad are nutritionally sound accompaniments.

If you include meat in your dinner, thaw it in a microwave oven or overnight in the refrigerator. The microwave is perhaps the cook's most important time-saving device. Microwaving vegetables saves time and preserves nutrients because it requires minimal water and discourages overcooking. A microwave oven is also useful for heating up leftovers.

When you have time to cook, cook for an army and freeze the leftovers. Chili, soup, and spaghetti sauce freeze well and sometimes improve in flavor after being frozen and reheated. All casseroles, including lasagna, can be divided into single- or family-sized portions and frozen for weeks until needed.

Foods prepared ahead of time in this way can provide the focal point for your meal. And fixing a vegetable or warming a loaf of bread to accompany a hearty soup is not nearly as overwhelming as starting a meal from scratch.

COLD FOOD SAFETY TIPS

Refrigerate foods such as hard-cooked eggs, meat, milk, and milk products (and salads that contain them) until just before you leave home. It is important to keep cold foods at refrigerator temperature. These suggestions will help you keep your "brown bag" lunch cold until you are ready to eat it.

♦ Use a vacuum bottle for foods that need to be kept cold, such as milk and yogurt.
♦ Purchase an insulated lunch box for your food rather than use a paper bag.
♦ Include an ice pack or freezer pack in your lunch box.
♦ Freeze your sandwich and pack it frozen.
♦ Store your lunch in a refrigerator, if available.

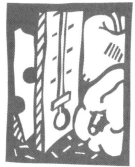

FOOD STORAGE AND PREPARATION

ALL FOODS DETERIORATE WITH TIME, some of them far more rapidly than others. Maintaining food in the freshest state possible is important to avoid contamination and receive the food's maximum nutritional value. By using appropriate food storage and preparation methods you can keep your food safe and the loss of nutrients to a minimum.

Bacterial decomposition
Bacteria (and fungi) use all forms of dead plant and animal matter as a source of energy. They gain the energy by oxidizing the carbon compounds of the organic matter, releasing carbon dioxide in the process. Some bacteria release ammonia or hydrogen sulfide, which accounts for the unpleasant smell of many decaying animal foods, such as eggs and fish (below).

The substances we eat as food are almost all of organic origin – that is, they were once part of a living organism. Even artificial foods such as soft drinks usually contain a vegetable base. Most foods are subject to decomposition and decay. The storage and preparation methods recommended on these pages can only slow down or arrest spoilage for variable amounts of time.

FOOD DETERIORATION

The agents that cause foods to decay are bacteria, fungi, loss of or exposure to moisture, sunlight, and certain enzymes contained within the food. The action of each of these agents is affected by ambient temperature. Deep freezing, for example, completely stops not only the activity of all microbes but also the action of the food's own enzymes. Heating to a high temperature (which is done during the pasteurization of milk) kills any disease-causing microorganisms with which the food is contaminated. Other factors, such as whether the food is exposed to air, also affect the rate at which food spoilage occurs.

The enzymes involved in the process of decay become active when the food is harvested or slaughtered. Even so, many

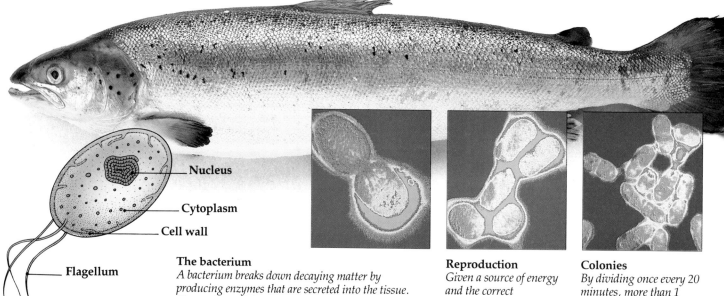

Nucleus

Cytoplasm

Cell wall

Flagellum

The bacterium
A bacterium breaks down decaying matter by producing enzymes that are secreted into the tissue. The products of the enzymatic action are soluble organic compounds such as amino acids, which can be absorbed through the cell wall and used as energy.

Reproduction
Given a source of energy and the correct temperature, bacteria reproduce by a process of cell division.

Colonies
By dividing once every 20 minutes, more than 1 million bacteria can be produced in 7 hours from a single bacterium.

foods, especially root crops and some fruits, remain fresh for months in good storage conditions.

The deterioration process, once started, is encouraged by enzymes that work in different ways. Some enzymes cause the destruction of certain nutrients by promoting oxidation, although oxidation can occur more slowly without enzymes being present. The browning of food tissues is also caused by enzyme activity. Finally, enzymes are involved in the ripening of fruits and vegetables. It is the activity of enzymes, converting starches to sugars, that causes a banana to change from green to yellow to brown.

There is no precise moment at which a food suddenly becomes inedible. There is, rather, a gradual deterioration, and the human palate is usually most comfortable with a particular stage in the continuum from ripening to decay. In general, you can trust your senses of smell and taste to exclude food that has gone bad. However, remember that certain contaminants of food, such as salmonella and staphylococcal bacteria, are odorless and tasteless.

STORAGE

The storage lives of different foods vary considerably. There are no hard and fast rules about the storage life of any food. The length of time a food remains fresh depends largely on the initial quality of the food, as well as on temperature, packaging, and moisture content. Most packaged foods are labeled with storage recommendations and many have "sell-by" dates printed on the packaging.

Microorganisms multiply at a much slower rate if the storage temperature of food is 40°F (5°C) or below. Meat, eggs, dairy products, and other perishables should be stored at this temperature. Meat and poultry may be stored in their original wrapping for about 2 days in the refrigerator. For slightly longer storage, wrap meat loosely in plastic wrap.

HOW LONG SHOULD FOODS LAST?

The food storage times given below are conservative estimates. The life of any food depends on its freshness and the conditions under which it is stored. High-quality food stored under ideal conditions can usually be kept for longer periods.

FROZEN FOODS	TIME Months
Bread	3
Fish	2 to 3
Fruit	12
Fruit juice	12
Ice cream	2
Meat	6
Vegetables	6

FOODS IN CANS AND JARS	TIME Months
Baby foods	6
Beer	3
Fish	12
Fruit	12
Fruit juice	6
Meat	12
Soft drinks	3
Soup	12
Vege-tables	6

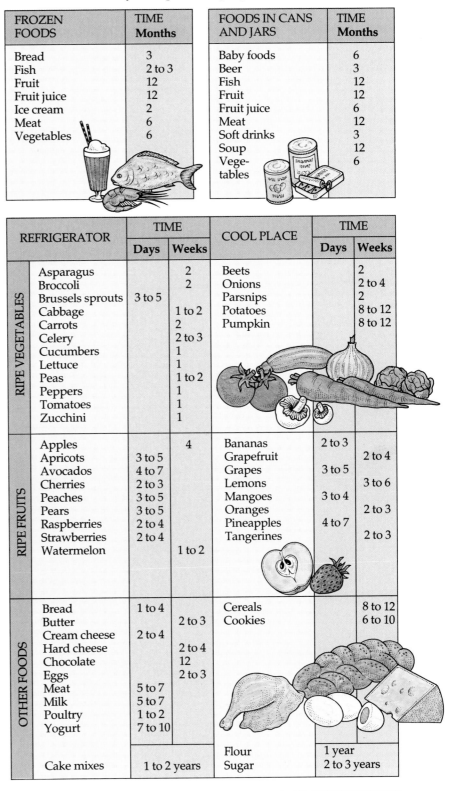

REFRIGERATOR		TIME Days	TIME Weeks	COOL PLACE	TIME Days	TIME Weeks
RIPE VEGETABLES	Asparagus		2	Beets		2
	Broccoli		2	Onions		2 to 4
	Brussels sprouts	3 to 5		Parsnips		2
	Cabbage		1 to 2	Potatoes		8 to 12
	Carrots		2	Pumpkin		8 to 12
	Celery		2 to 3			
	Cucumbers		1			
	Lettuce		1			
	Peas		1 to 2			
	Peppers		1			
	Tomatoes		1			
	Zucchini		1			
RIPE FRUITS	Apples		4	Bananas	2 to 3	
	Apricots	3 to 5		Grapefruit		2 to 4
	Avocados	4 to 7		Grapes	3 to 5	
	Cherries	2 to 3		Lemons		3 to 6
	Peaches	3 to 5		Mangoes	3 to 4	
	Pears	3 to 5		Oranges		2 to 3
	Raspberries	2 to 4		Pineapples	4 to 7	
	Strawberries	2 to 4		Tangerines		2 to 3
	Watermelon		1 to 2			
OTHER FOODS	Bread	1 to 4		Cereals		8 to 12
	Butter		2 to 3	Cookies		6 to 10
	Cream cheese	2 to 4				
	Hard cheese		2 to 4			
	Chocolate		12			
	Eggs		2 to 3			
	Meat	5 to 7				
	Milk	5 to 7				
	Poultry	1 to 2				
	Yogurt	7 to 10				
	Cake mixes	1 to 2 years		Flour	1 year	
				Sugar	2 to 3 years	

COOKING UTENSILS

Cooking pots and pans manufactured from enameled iron, steel, stainless steel, glass, and some earthenware release very little material into food during the cooking process. Aluminum migrates from utensils into food, especially when the metal is exposed to highly acidic foods such as tomatoes, vinegar, and citrus fruits. Most of the aluminum that is taken into the body is excreted. The remainder is stored in the lungs, brain, liver, and thyroid gland. Some studies report an increased amount of aluminum in the brains of people who have Alzheimer's disease. However, there is no conclusive evidence that aluminum is a causative factor.

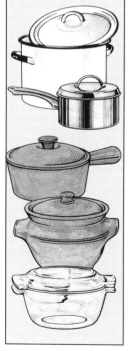

The temperature of your freezer should be 0°F (-18°C). A freezer thermometer will help you monitor any variation in temperature. Wrap fresh meats tightly in aluminum foil, plastic wrap, or freezer paper, date them, and use the oldest packages first. Wrap other foods tightly or seal them in covered plastic containers for freezer storage.

COOKING

Cooking tenderizes many foods, making them easier to chew and swallow. In some cases, cooking enhances the flavor and makes the foods we eat more appetizing. Cooking also makes some foods easier to digest, an important consideration with starchy foods such as potatoes. Heat destroys natural toxins such as those contained in lentils. It also kills harmful microorganisms that lead to undesirable flavors and illness.

Cooking methods

The method you choose for cooking a food depends on several factors, including the food to be cooked, the equipment and time available to you, and individual preference.

Heat can be applied to food in three different ways. Direct heat may be used, with or without the addition of fat, as in roasting, grilling, baking, and microwave cooking. Heat may be applied through water, with or without additional ingredients (such as wine, salt, and sugar), as in boiling, steaming, and stewing. And the heat may be conducted through oil, as in stir-frying.

Nutrient losses during cooking

The loss of protein and carbohydrates during cooking is generally small and unimportant. The amount of fat in the food may be increased or decreased, depending on the cooking method used

WAYS OF MINIMIZING NUTRIENT LOSSES

 When you shop for produce, choose fresh fruits and vegetables carefully. Avoid purchasing foods that have bruises or cuts or that look as if they might be old and past their peak.

 Wash fresh fruits and vegetables under cold, running water using a little dishwashing liquid. Soap may help remove the residue of stubborn fat-soluble pesticides. Rinse all produce throughly. Do not soak fruits and vegetables in still water for any length of time or nutrients may pass into the water.

 If possible, cook the food whole. If you have to slice or chop food, keep the pieces as large as possible so as to keep their surface area to a minimum. The greater the surface area, the greater the loss of water-soluble vitamins by leaching.

 Try to make salads just before eating them. Fruits and vegetables that are cut up in advance and left exposed to air lose vitamins.

 When boiling, put raw food in boiling, not cold, water. When you can, steam the food rather than boil it. If you have a microwave oven, cook vegetables and fruits in it using little or no water. Any leftover water contains water-soluble vitamins and minerals and can be used in soups.

 Cook food for the shortest time possible. Eat it as soon as you can and do not keep the food hot for prolonged periods. If you thaw frozen fish or vegetables before cooking, cook them immediately. Keeping them at warm temperatures after thawing allows rapid multiplication of microbes.

and whether or not you add fat in the process. In general, any method that allows the fat to drain during cooking decreases the amount of fat in the food.

The vitamins lost in the greatest quantities during cooking are vitamin C and folic acid and, to a lesser extent, thiamine and other B-complex vitamins, such as vitamin B_6. These are the most heat-sensitive vitamins. They are destroyed by heat and are also sensitive to prolonged cooking times and being kept warm for long periods.

Vitamin C, iron, and the B-complex vitamins are also lost in significant amounts when foods containing them are cooked in water, especially during boiling. The loss of water-soluble nutrients increases correspondingly to the amount of water used in the cooking process. Steaming and microwave cooking reduce the loss of nutrients because the food does not always come into direct contact with the water.

Pressure-cooking involves high temperatures for shorter times. It retains more nutrients than conventional boiling, though food that is steamed or boiled in a small amount of water in a tightly covered pan or microwaved is likely to be as nutritious.

HIGH for 1 minute. If the water becomes hot, the dish is suitable; if the dish becomes hot, it isn't.

Plastic wraps designed for use in a microwave oven are useful for covering containers to hold the heat — usually in the form of steam — in check. Both dishes with covers and dishes covered with plastic wrap may feel cool to the touch when removed from the microwave oven. Be extremely cautious when you remove the lid or plastic wrap. The steam inside the container can easily scald your hand or arm.

> **WARNING**
>
> The newest pacemaker models are not affected by any microwaves that may "leak" from your microwave oven. However, the older pacemakers are vulnerable to microwaves. If you have a pacemaker, ask your doctor for advice.

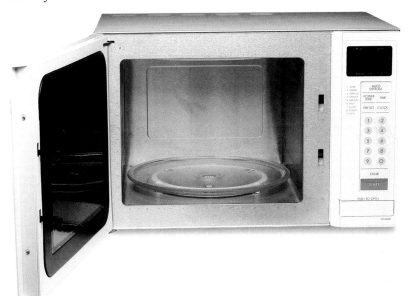

USING A MICROWAVE

A microwave oven works by passing microwave energy into the cavity of the oven. The oven walls and base deflect the microwaves into the food. This causes the molecules of water in the food to vibrate. The vibration causes friction, which produces heat.

Any material (such as paper) through which microwaves will pass is suitable for use in a microwave oven. Do not use metal cooking utensils or foil. Most basic cookware can be used in a microwave. If you are in doubt about whether a cooking dish is suitable, test the dish by placing about a cup of water in a glass cup inside the dish. Microwave on

THE ADVANTAGES OF MICROWAVE COOKING	
Nutritional value	Many people find that they are less likely to overcook foods. As a result, foods retain more vitamins and minerals.
Flavor and color	Flavors are not impaired, and vegetables remain crisp and brightly colored if not overcooked.
Low fat	Foods can be cooked without adding any fat or with very little fat.
Safety	The oven stays cool during cooking, so you are less likely to burn yourself. However, be sure to read the safety tips in your instruction booklet.
Cooking smells	Cooking times are shorter, so cooking odors are dramatically reduced.
Speed	You can save between one half and two thirds of the normal cooking times for many foods.
Economy	Faster cooking times mean lower utility costs.

MYTH AND REALITY

Every day we read contradictory advice about our diets. When faced with conflicting information, many people rely in the end on their personal beliefs about nutrition or on the recommendations of others. Our views about the values of foods can be distorted by our wish to discover miracle cures for common ailments or our longing to find that the food we enjoy is, in fact, "good" for us. Here are some common myths about food that may have reached you through TV or magazine reports or may have been passed on by relatives and friends.

Do carrots help you see in the dark?
Eating carrots will improve your vision only if you have difficulty adjusting to the dark because of a deficiency of vitamin A. Night blindness is one of the symptoms caused by vitamin A deficiency, and carrots are a good source of vitamin A. However, people who are in good health and eat a well-balanced diet gain nothing from increasing their vitamin A intake above the normal recommendations. Neither carrots nor vitamins can improve the night vision of well-nourished people.

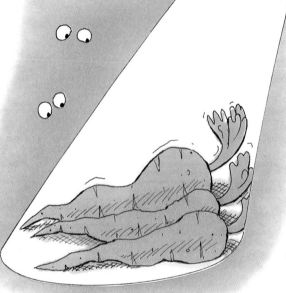

Are there any specific foods that can help you lose weight?
No. Perhaps the idea is fostered by fad diets, many of which are based on a single food, such as grapefruit, or on a small number of foods. Grapefruit, celery, and foods like them are useful constituents of a healthy diet because they are low in calories, contain little or no fat, contribute some vitamins and minerals, and are often also high in fiber. However, the best way to lose weight is to increase your energy expenditure and to eat less.

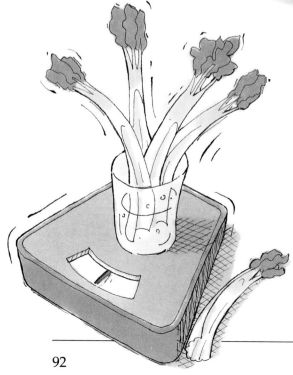

Can foods labeled "cholesterol-free" raise my cholesterol level?
Yes. Just because a bag of potato chips is labeled "cholesterol-free" doesn't mean that it can't raise your cholesterol level. Almost all saturated fats can drive up your cholesterol level, so it's important to think about how much saturated fat (the fats that are solid at room temperature) you eat. Remember that if you are concerned about your cholesterol level, you should reduce your intake of all fats, not only cholesterol-containing foods.

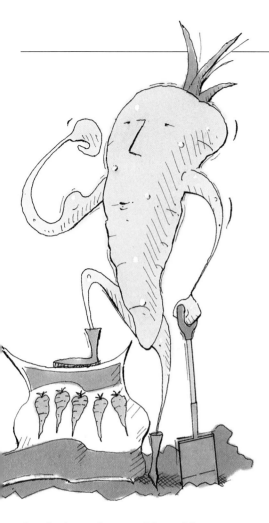

Is it true that brown sugar is better for you than white?

White sugar, which is refined, contains no nutrients other than sucrose. Because brown sugar is not refined to the degree that white is, it retains greater amounts of minerals and vitamins. However, these amounts are far too small in proportion to the high calorie content of the sugar to warrant the extolling of brown sugar as an essential nutrient source. Possibly because nutrition experts recommend brown whole-grain bread and brown, whole-grain rice, the belief has grown that all brown foods are good for us.

Are fruits and vegetables without pesticides and preservatives better for you than conventionally produced ones?

Not necessarily. It would be ideal for everyone to eat freshly picked fruits and vegetables; they contain the most vitamins and are less likely to be spoiled by bacteria or molds, some of which may be harmful. All food begins to spoil after a day or two of storage, so the food industry uses chemical preservatives, freezing, drying, and other methods to delay this process. In fact, some of the molds in food are more harmful to humans than the preservatives used to combat them. In addition, crops that are not sprayed with pesticides are more vulnerable to a variety of insects and other pests. Unless we are able to eat truly fresh food from a garden or a local farm, it is probably worth treating food to maintain wholesomeness and keep costs down.

Is snacking between meals bad for your health?

That depends on the snack. Nutritious snacks planned as part of your day's food can help you meet your nutrient needs. Plan ahead to make each snack something you like that is nutritious, too. Try to choose snacks that are lower in fat, cholesterol, sugar, and salt than the standard "junk" items. Or make adjustments for the extra fat, sugar, and sodium in a favorite snack by reducing the amount of these substances in other foods you eat that day. If you like to munch all day, pack a lunch that includes items such as a lean-meat sandwich, fruit, and yogurt and snack periodically throughout your day.

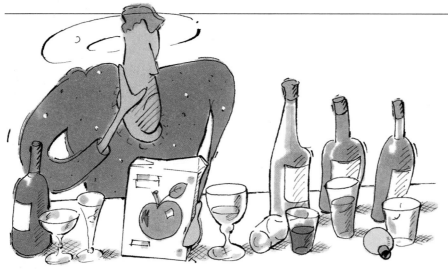

Is fish really "brain food"?
No. Although fish is a highly nutritious and valuable food, the brain functions just as effectively on a well-balanced vegetarian or meat diet as on one containing fish. This myth, like the spinach myth, probably dates back to attempts by parents to persuade reluctant children to eat foods they believed were especially good for them.

Is apple juice good for a hangover?
Yes, but only to the extent that a hangover can be improved by drinking plenty of any nonalcoholic fluids to replace fluids lost by the diuretic effect of alcohol. Nonalcoholic beverages may also help relieve the unpleasant taste in the mouth experienced by many people after heavy drinking. However, there is no miracle ingredient in apple juice – or in any other hangover "cure" – that can immediately restore the health of a person who has drunk too much. If you develop a hangover, rest quietly while the hangover symptoms gradually disappear. And, while you're resting, consider why you have a hangover in the first place. Drinking enough alcohol to produce a hangover is not good for you.

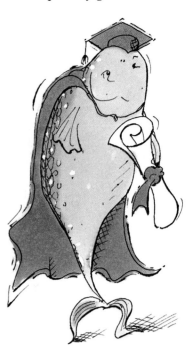

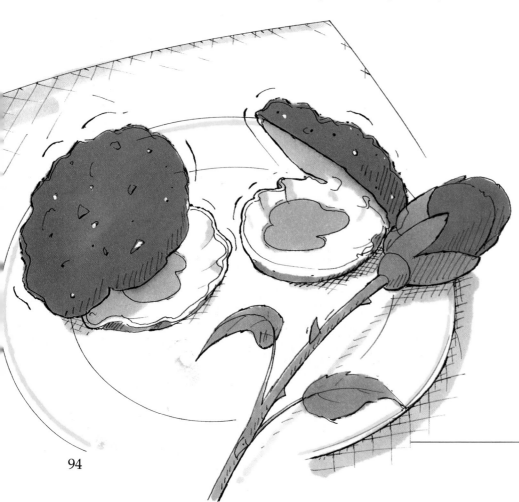

Are oysters an aphrodisiac?
No. Over the centuries, various substances, including ginger, ginseng, marijuana, tigers' whiskers, and oysters, have earned a reputation as aphrodisiacs – substances capable of increasing sexual drive and enhancing sexual performance. No substance has been proven to have an aphrodisiac effect. Some, such as Spanish fly (a powder made from dried beetles), have caused serious side effects and even death. It is worth noting, however, that, if a person strongly believes a food or other substance has an aphrodisiac effect, then it may have such an effect, but only because of the power of suggestion, rather than any known physical effect.

Does an apple a day really keep the doctor away?

A medium-sized apple consists of about 50 percent water and contains about 40 kilocalories, 3 grams of fiber, 3 milligrams of vitamin C, and small amounts of iron, thiamine, and niacin. The idea that eating an apple a day can guarantee good health is a myth. However, as a way of suggesting that we eat fresh fruit each day, it has real value. Eating plenty of fruit is one way to obtain adequate fiber, vitamins, and minerals. A piece of fruit also makes a good low-calorie snack.

Is it true that the green part of potatoes is poisonous and dangerous to eat?

Green potatoes or green parts of a potato may contain small amounts of solanine, a chemical substance that makes potatoes bitter and indigestible. It is advisable to avoid eating the solanine by cutting out any green parts from potatoes before cooking. However, green potatoes would have to be consumed in enormous amounts ever to result in serious poisoning.

Does spinach make you strong?

One of our childhood cartoons showed a muscular sailor magically improving his strength by swallowing a can of spinach. There is, however, no medical basis for this idea. Some children were forced to eat spinach during the 1950s in the belief that it would be especially good for them. Spinach is certainly a good source of vitamins A and C and of the minerals iron and copper, but it is no more or less nutritious than other green leafy vegetables.

CHAPTER FOUR

DIET AND YOUR WEIGHT

OST PEOPLE NEED little encouragement to "eat, drink, and be merry." In addition, enjoying food is a sign of a healthy appetite and a readiness to appreciate an important aspect of the earth's bounty. In today's sedentary society, the pleasure we derive from food makes it easy to continue eating far beyond what we need to fulfill our body's needs. The result is that all the calories that we don't "burn off" through exercise are stored in the body as fat. Food intake and body weight are modified by a host of factors, the most important of which is the amount of energy you expend through activity. In this chapter we examine the relationship between exercise, what you eat, and your weight.

For several decades the overwhelming message brought to us by the media has been that you must be thin to have self-esteem and to be attractive. In the 1990s, this message is being replaced by the realization that maintaining your body at the level at which it functions best (and at its optimum weight) is a vital safeguard against premature illness. Being overweight is a significant factor in the development of life-threatening diseases such as coronary heart disease and some cancers.

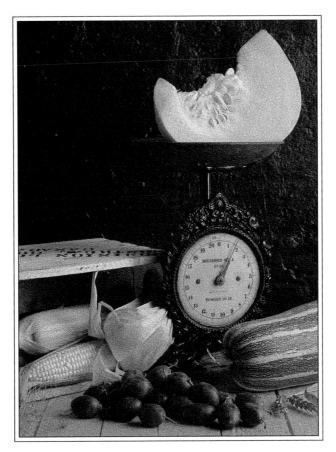

The first section of this chapter, WEIGHT GAIN AND OBESITY, shows you how to determine your ideal weight and explains why many people gain weight, sometimes becoming obese, despite efforts to control it. It also explains how energy needs vary. Finally, it reviews the influence of genes and family eating patterns on weight.

Most people must cope with being overweight at some point in their lives. In the second section, LOSING WEIGHT, we describe methods of weight loss that are safe, achievable, and most likely to keep the weight off. The vital role that exercise plays in long-term weight loss is highlighted, and popular diets are analyzed for their strong and weak points. In cases of extreme obesity, some people resort to dramatic measures of weight control, such as drugs, jaw wiring, and stomach operations. These techniques are evaluated.

If obesity lies at one end of the weight spectrum, the starvation and binge-purge disorders of ANOREXIA NERVOSA AND BULIMIA lie at the other. The final section in this chapter addresses the physical and psychological effects of these two conditions. It also describes the forms of treatment that people have undergone to restore themselves to a healthy weight.

WEIGHT GAIN AND OBESITY

IT IS ESTIMATED THAT about one quarter of the US population carries too much fat. At least 30 million Americans are seriously overweight and the number is growing. Between 5 and 10 percent of our children are obese. Weight problems are taking a toll on the health of the nation, and healthier eating habits and life-styles must be established if the pattern is not to persist in future generations.

Are you overweight?
If you weigh more than the upper limit of the ranges given below, you are probably overweight. If you weigh more than 20 percent more than the upper limit, you are obese. Being overweight and being obese are not synonymous. Obesity occurs when your proportion of body fat is too high.

Several factors that govern your body weight are beyond your control – height, sex, and general type of build. Weight tables offer guidelines to help you determine whether you are underweight, of normal weight, or overweight.

Normal weight is traditionally defined as a weight that falls within the ranges given in the chart below (the figures are for unclothed weight and for height without shoes). According to the Metropolitan Life Insurance Company, a weight that lies within these ranges offers the greatest life expectancy for each of the combinations of gender, height, and frame.

HOW MUCH SHOULD YOU WEIGH?

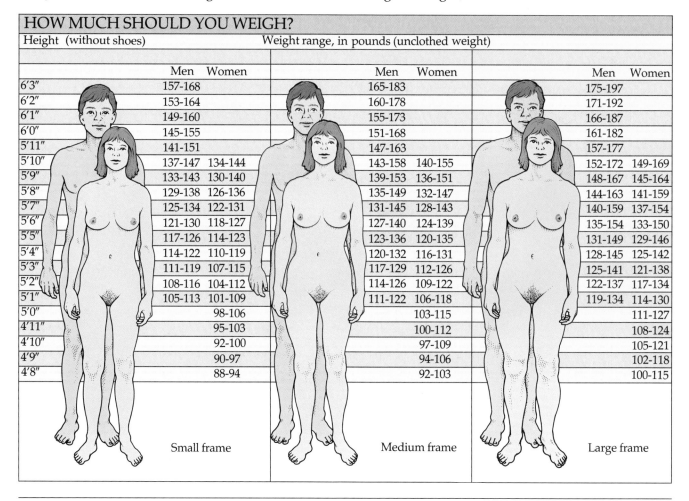

Height (without shoes)	Weight range, in pounds (unclothed weight)					
	Men	Women	Men	Women	Men	Women
6'3"	157-168		165-183		175-197	
6'2"	153-164		160-178		171-192	
6'1"	149-160		155-173		166-187	
6'0"	145-155		151-168		161-182	
5'11"	141-151		147-163		157-177	
5'10"	137-147	134-144	143-158	140-155	152-172	149-169
5'9"	133-143	130-140	139-153	136-151	148-167	145-164
5'8"	129-138	126-136	135-149	132-147	144-163	141-159
5'7"	125-134	122-131	131-145	128-143	140-159	137-154
5'6"	121-130	118-127	127-140	124-139	135-154	133-150
5'5"	117-126	114-123	123-136	120-135	131-149	129-146
5'4"	114-122	110-119	120-132	116-131	128-145	125-142
5'3"	111-119	107-115	117-129	112-126	125-141	121-138
5'2"	108-116	104-112	114-126	109-122	122-137	117-134
5'1"	105-113	101-109	111-122	106-118	119-134	114-130
5'0"		98-106		103-115		111-127
4'11"		95-103		100-112		108-124
4'10"		92-100		97-109		105-121
4'9"		90-97		94-106		102-118
4'8"		88-94		92-103		100-115

Small frame — Medium frame — Large frame

UNDERSTANDING BODY WEIGHT

In adult life, the weight of your skeleton and internal organs remains almost constant; any changes in body weight are caused by variations in the amount of water, muscle, or fat.

Changes in your body's water balance can add or subtract from 1 to 5 pounds over short periods of time. Fluctuations occur as hormone levels change and with perspiration. The weight of your muscles increases in response to regular hard exercise and decreases during prolonged rest or immobilization. All fat is energy stored against future needs in case food is not available.

Obesity

Obesity is strictly defined not as excessive weight, but as an excessive amount of body fat in relation to the rest of the body. In healthy young adult men, about 15 to 20 percent of body weight consists of fat. In healthy young adult women, the percentage is higher – about 20 to 25 percent.

FOOD CONSUMPTION AND ENERGY EXPENDITURE

Your body weight remains more or less stable only if the energy content of your food intake is balanced by your total energy expenditure. If you take in fewer calories or if your energy expenditure rises, you will tend to lose weight. If you take in more food or if your energy expenditure drops, the surplus energy is laid down as fat. Fat allows the body to store the maximum amount of energy in the minimum amount of space. It is important to remember that your body's water content, the major component of body weight, is regulated independently of energy expenditure.

Active people who are recuperating from injury or illness in bed may gain

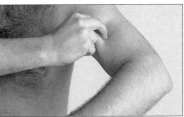

Front of arm

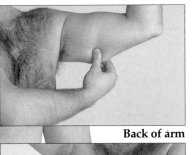

Back of arm

Waist

Shoulder blade

weight if their food intake remains at its former level. Similarly, athletes are prone to obesity when they retire. In contrast, an overweight, sedentary person who begins to walk briskly for about 1½ miles every day (without any increase in food intake) will eventually lose weight. This is because the energy in that person's food will not be sufficient to cover energy expenditure, and the balance will be drawn from fat reserves.

Individual variations

There is substantial variation in the amount of energy that different people require from food to maintain their body weight at its optimum level. This is partly because of variations in the amount of physical exercise each person gets – people who are very active need more energy than do those who are sedentary. Even more important, energy requirements vary due to an individual's basal metabolic rate. Two people of the same age, sex, and weight can have different basal metabolic rates.

How is obesity measured?
One approximate method of assessing how much body fat you are carrying is to pinch a fold of skin between finger and thumb at the waist (and over the abdomen), at the shoulder blade, and at the upper part of the arm (front and back) as shown above. Be sure not to include any muscle when you pinch. Skinfolds thicker than 1 inch suggest you would benefit from losing weight. For more accurate medical assessment, a fold of skin is pinched and grasped with standard pressure using calipers. The thickness of the fold is registered on a dial and tables are used to convert the readings into percentages of body fat.

MONITOR YOUR SYMPTOMS
EXCESS WEIGHT IN ADULTS

Being overweight is a serious hazard to your health, increasing the risk of high blood pressure, coronary heart disease, diabetes, and other disorders, and aggravating any existing arthritis. If your weight exceeds what is recommended for your sex, height, and build (see the table on page 98), follow the chart below to determine why. Weight gain is often caused simply by eating too much or by being inactive but, in some cases, there is a medical reason.

KEY FACTORS IN WEIGHT LOSS
◆ Cut down on high-calorie beverages, such as alcohol
◆ Limit your intake of foods high in fat and sugar
◆ Eat five small meals throughout the day
◆ Use low-fat dairy products
◆ Eat more high-fiber foods
◆ Exercise regularly

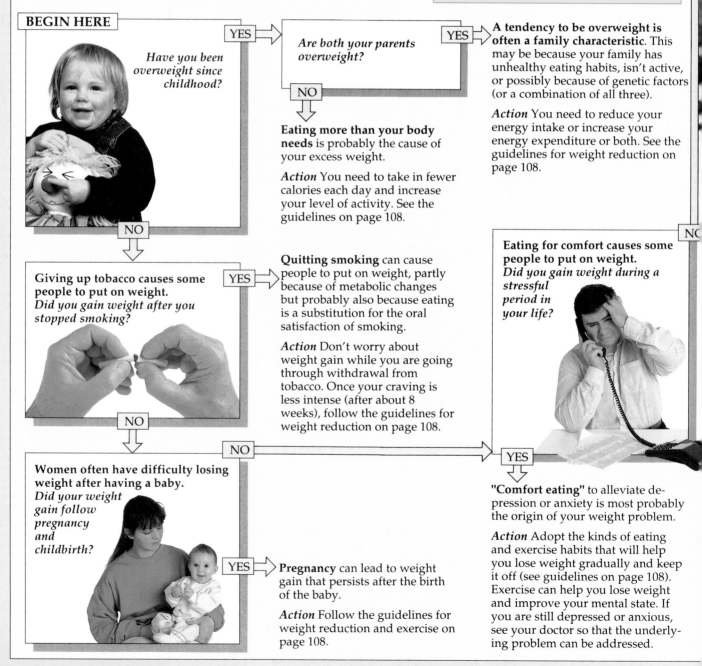

BEGIN HERE

Have you been overweight since childhood? — YES →

Are both your parents overweight? — YES →

A tendency to be overweight is often a family characteristic. This may be because your family has unhealthy eating habits, isn't active, or possibly because of genetic factors (or a combination of all three).

Action You need to reduce your energy intake or increase your energy expenditure or both. See the guidelines for weight reduction on page 108.

NO ↓

Eating more than your body needs is probably the cause of your excess weight.

Action You need to take in fewer calories each day and increase your level of activity. See the guidelines on page 108.

NO ↓

Giving up tobacco causes some people to put on weight.
Did you gain weight after you stopped smoking? — YES →

Quitting smoking can cause people to put on weight, partly because of metabolic changes but probably also because eating is a substitution for the oral satisfaction of smoking.

Action Don't worry about weight gain while you are going through withdrawal from tobacco. Once your craving is less intense (after about 8 weeks), follow the guidelines for weight reduction on page 108.

Eating for comfort causes some people to put on weight.
Did you gain weight during a stressful period in your life?

NO ↓

Women often have difficulty losing weight after having a baby.
Did your weight gain follow pregnancy and childbirth?

NO →

YES ↓

"Comfort eating" to alleviate depression or anxiety is most probably the origin of your weight problem.

Action Adopt the kinds of eating and exercise habits that will help you lose weight gradually and keep it off (see guidelines on page 108). Exercise can help you lose weight and improve your mental state. If you are still depressed or anxious, see your doctor so that the underlying problem can be addressed.

YES →

Pregnancy can lead to weight gain that persists after the birth of the baby.

Action Follow the guidelines for weight reduction and exercise on page 108.

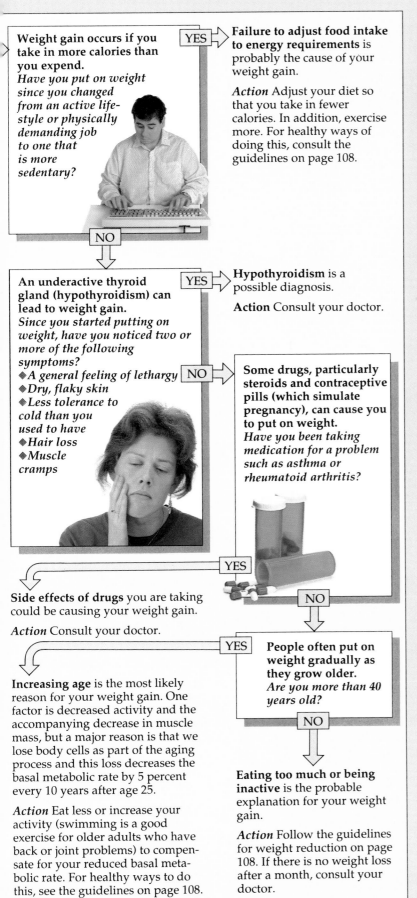

Weight gain occurs if you take in more calories than you expend.
Have you put on weight since you changed from an active life-style or physically demanding job to one that is more sedentary?

| YES |

Failure to adjust food intake to energy requirements is probably the cause of your weight gain.

Action Adjust your diet so that you take in fewer calories. In addition, exercise more. For healthy ways of doing this, consult the guidelines on page 108.

| NO |

An underactive thyroid gland (hypothyroidism) can lead to weight gain.
Since you started putting on weight, have you noticed two or more of the following symptoms?
◆ *A general feeling of lethargy*
◆ *Dry, flaky skin*
◆ *Less tolerance to cold than you used to have*
◆ *Hair loss*
◆ *Muscle cramps*

| YES |

Hypothyroidism is a possible diagnosis.

Action Consult your doctor.

| NO |

Some drugs, particularly steroids and contraceptive pills (which simulate pregnancy), can cause you to put on weight.
Have you been taking medication for a problem such as asthma or rheumatoid arthritis?

| YES |

Side effects of drugs you are taking could be causing your weight gain.

Action Consult your doctor.

| NO |

Increasing age is the most likely reason for your weight gain. One factor is decreased activity and the accompanying decrease in muscle mass, but a major reason is that we lose body cells as part of the aging process and this loss decreases the basal metabolic rate by 5 percent every 10 years after age 25.

Action Eat less or increase your activity (swimming is a good exercise for older adults who have back or joint problems) to compensate for your reduced basal metabolic rate. For healthy ways to do this, see the guidelines on page 108.

| YES |

People often put on weight gradually as they grow older.
Are you more than 40 years old?

| NO |

Eating too much or being inactive is the probable explanation for your weight gain.

Action Follow the guidelines for weight reduction on page 108. If there is no weight loss after a month, consult your doctor.

BASAL METABOLIC RATE

The basal metabolic rate is the energy required to maintain at rest the basic functions of the body, such as breathing, body temperature, and heart rate. Since the cells of your body are responsible for basal metabolism, the basal metabolic rate is proportional to the number of cells, particularly the number of muscle cells. Your basal metabolic rate changes dramatically with age as lean body mass is lost. The basal metabolic rate is about one quarter less at age 75 than it is at age 25. This is an important idea since one of the benefits of exercise may be to slow the age-related loss of lean body mass by increasing your muscle mass, thus preventing weight gain with age from a declining basal metabolic rate.

Low basal metabolic rate

A person with a low metabolic rate requires fewer calories to supply his or her energy needs than a person of the same sex, age, and weight who has the same level of physical activity but a higher metabolic rate. If two people have identical levels of energy intake and physical activity, one may gain weight and the other may not, simply because one has a lower, more efficient, metabolic rate. This observation has led to the use of the term "underburners" to describe people with low metabolic rates.

High basal metabolic rate

Individuals with a higher basal metabolic rate (sometimes called "overburners") are usually able to consume quantities of calories normally considered excessive without becoming obese.

Smoking and basal metabolic rate

Tobacco smoking can slightly raise the metabolic rate, while decreasing appetite. Quitting smoking can slightly lower the rate, while restoring the appetite. However, it is always better to quit smoking, even if you gain some weight, than it is to continue smoking.

WHAT ARE THE RISKS OF OBESITY?

In general, overweight people do not live as long as people of normal weight. The increased death rate is due to three groups of diseases – circulatory system diseases, such as hypertension (high blood pressure), coronary heart disease, and stroke; diabetes, which predisposes a person to atherosclerosis; and digestive system disease, especially gallbladder disease. In addition to these risks, overweight people are prone to other disorders.

Breathlessness
Obesity may cause breathlessness by interfering with the movement of the diaphragm and by increasing the workload of the heart.

Gallstones
Obesity causes an increase in the synthesis of cholesterol in the liver and in the amount of cholesterol excreted in the bile. The result is an increased precipitation of cholesterol crystals in the form of gallstones.

Osteoarthritis
Excess weight in a person with osteoarthritis means the diseased joints must bear more weight. The relationship of obesity in causing osteoarthritis is not known.

Cancer
The relation between obesity and a higher incidence of cancer of the colon, breast, uterus, gallbladder, and stomach (see DIET AND CANCER on page 128) has been noted in various population studies and awaits further confirmation.

Varicose veins
Varicose veins are a problem for obese people, in whom the accompanying immobility aggravates the varicose veins.

Coronary heart disease
Men who carry their extra weight in the abdomen, or paunch, are more likely to have coronary heart disease than men who carry the extra weight elsewhere. Men who are 15 to 25 percent overweight have a 30 percent higher risk of dying of this cause. Men who are 50 percent overweight have a 50 percent higher mortality from heart attack, and men more than 60 percent overweight have an 80 percent increase in mortality.

Backache
If the upper part of the body is heavy and lacking in muscle tone, pressure is placed on the lower part of the spine, resulting in backache.

Hypertension
Men 5 to 15 percent overweight have an increased mortality of 70 percent and men more than 15 percent overweight are two and a half times as likely to die of the effects of hypertension as men of normal weight and comparable age. Modest reductions in weight can have a significant effect on lowering blood pressure.

Intertrigo
Obesity causes skin-to-skin contact (intertrigo) in such areas as the breast and chest, abdomen, and upper part of the thighs. Friction during activity, particularly in warm weather, may cause chafing and fungal infections.

Diabetes
Diabetics who are 5 to 15 percent overweight have an increased mortality of 25 percent. Those who are 15 to 25 percent overweight have twice the death rate at any age. Diabetics who are more than 25 percent overweight have five times the normal death rate.

TOO MANY CALORIES

A common explanation for weight gain in certain people is that they consume certain foods, sometimes in large quantities, without realizing that the foods have a high calorie content. Alcoholic drinks contain many calories, but because they are beverages their calorie content is often not appreciated. The same is true for sugar-rich, carbonated beverages. Potato chips and other snacks also contain "hidden" calories in the form of fat.

In developed countries, a more sedentary life-style can lead to obesity, whether by overeating or simply by exceeding the balance between energy intake and output. Many people whose hunger is satisfied by eating dinner are still able to find room for more food of a different kind, such as a bowl of ice cream. Overeating is also encouraged by the availability of high-calorie snacks, candy, cakes, alcohol, and soft drinks.

High-energy foods

The high energy density of much of today's food is another factor that contributes to weight gain and obesity. An energy-dense food is any food that is rich in calories per unit weight. The illustration below shows four foods, each of which contains 250 kilocalories. You can keep your weight under control by eating foods that have a low energy density. Low energy-dense foods, such as potatoes or rice without added fat, often have a high fiber content as well.

Energy-dense foods, such as fats or refined carbohydrates, on the other hand, provide large quantities of calories in a small volume. You may be inclined to eat much more of these foods before you begin to feel satisfied and full. Thus, a diet high in refined sugar, high-fat snack foods, and fats in general often leads to a much higher calorie intake than a diet consisting mainly of high-fiber sources such as fruits, vegetables, and legumes.

FAT AND EXERCISE

It is common for your energy intake (what you eat and drink) to exceed your energy expenditure (the amount you exercise). But how do you rectify the imbalance? Occasional bursts of activity are of limited value – walking a mile once, for example, uses up fewer than 100 kilocalories. However, if you walk that same mile every day, you will expend calories on a regular basis, increase your muscle mass (which increases your metabolic rate), mobilize your body fat, and depress your appetite.

WHAT IS ENERGY DENSITY?

All foods contain a specific amount of energy in a standard serving of a certain weight. If the energy yield of 100 grams of raw potatoes were measured in a laboratory, it would be substantially lower than the energy yield of 100 grams of butter. Thus, a potato is described as a low energy-dense food; butter is a high energy-dense food. Adding fat by frying a potato or using sour cream converts the potato into a high energy-dense food. All the foods shown at right contain 250 kilocalories. It is easier to exceed your energy requirements by eating a potato that has fat added than eating a potato on its own.

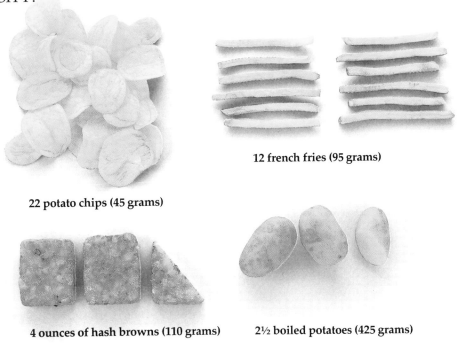

22 potato chips (45 grams)

12 french fries (95 grams)

4 ounces of hash browns (110 grams)

2½ boiled potatoes (425 grams)

WHERE ARE FAT DEPOSITS MOST LIKELY TO OCCUR?

Most fat is deposited immediately under the skin of the central zone of the body – around the waist, over the abdomen, over the buttock muscles, and under the skin of the breasts. Men and women have different fat distribution patterns. Men tend to accumulate fat in the abdominal area and women tend to accumulate it around the hips, thighs, and buttocks. Deposits of fat also occur under other areas of skin, such as the shoulders, arms, and legs. The shaded areas below show where fat can accumulate.

Omentum
It is common for obese people to have collections of fat inside the abdomen, mainly in the hanging fold of peritoneal membrane covering the intestines (the omentum) and against the inside of the back wall of the abdomen, around the kidneys.

Kidney

Fat

Omentum

Fat layer
The photograph at right shows the appearance of a layer of fat beneath the skin.

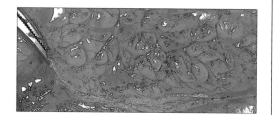

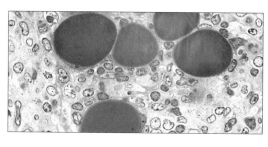

Fat cells
Magnified 800 times, the round cells here are adipocytes, or fat-storing cells.

LIFE-STYLE FACTORS

One of the most important contributing factors to becoming obese – even in children – is inactivity. Overeating by obese people is not as common as is a sedentary life-style. In some cases the way in which we respond to stress can be an underlying cause of obesity. Some people eat, often without appetite, as a "displacement activity." This means that, rather than cope with a stressful or emotional situation by confronting it (or the person who caused it), they eat.

Similarly, indulging in food or a particular type of food may serve as a substitute for an emotional need that is not being met. Food may also represent comfort in times of stress when there is no other solace (see EXCESS WEIGHT IN ADULTS on page 100). Just as excessive demands placed on some people may cause them to turn to food for comfort, a tedious, unstimulating life may have the same effect on others.

HORMONAL FACTORS

Hormonal disturbances can cause obesity, but only as part of recognizable medical syndromes, such as Cushing's syndrome, in which the pituitary gland and the adrenal glands malfunction. The appearance of a person with Cushing's syndrome is shown below. Thyroid underactivity accounts for only one case of obesity in 100. In spite of what many people believe, there is no common glandular cause for obesity.

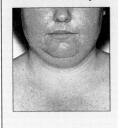

HEREDITY AND ENVIRONMENT

Many obese people have a family history of obesity. About 80 percent of obese children have an obese parent. In many cases, both parents are obese. Underweight parents rarely have overweight children and obese parents rarely have underweight children.

Researchers have suggested that a child's early habit of overeating, learned from his or her parents, may continue into adulthood. Alternatively, the excess energy intake may stimulate the production of fat cells, which persist into adulthood, leading to adult obesity. Other studies of obesity imply genetically based and difficult-to-detect individual differences in the ability to use calories even at rest. Many questions remain unanswered but there is little doubt that heredity plays an important role.

Prenatal influences

Obese women usually have larger babies than women of normal weight. Larger babies are often associated with complications during labor and delivery. Furthermore, diabetes often develops later in life in women who bear oversized babies. These facts suggest that environmental factors, such as a woman's nutritional status and, in turn, the nutrient supply to the fetus, can be important in determining long-term body size. Further evidence is supplied by the fact that twins who have very different body weights at birth tend to retain this difference throughout life. Parents are sometimes concerned that their babies are becoming too fat and will be obese later in life. There is no convincing evidence to support this notion. The risk of long-term obesity is greater with overweight teenagers, 80 percent of whom can be expected to be significantly overweight 30 years later. Only 20 percent of teenagers of normal weight become significantly overweight after 30 years.

ASK YOUR DOCTOR WEIGHT GAIN AND OBESITY

Q **My doctor tells me I should lose weight, but everyone in my family is big. Will dieting make any difference if I've inherited my size?**

A Families are usually overweight because the members share the same eating habits, such as a large breakfast every morning and the expectation of a dessert every evening. You may also share a dislike for exercise, an inactive life-style, or an inherited low basal metabolic rate. Any of these may lead to obesity. A controlled food intake or an increase in activity or both will help you achieve and maintain a healthful weight.

Q **My brother has convinced himself that he is obese because he has a glandular problem. Could he be right?**

A It is unlikely. Only one common glandular condition, hypothyroidism (underactivity of the thyroid gland), causes all the body processes to slow down, resulting in weight gain even during reduced calorie intake. However, hypothyroidism is rarely the cause of obesity.

Q **I am pregnant for the first time. Am I going to gain weight permanently?**

A Body fat that you gain during pregnancy need not persist, especially if you breast-feed, since milk production helps use up calories. When the fat does remain, it is usually because the woman is taking in calories that she no longer needs or because she gained excessive weight during pregnancy. With careful attention to calorie intake and regular exercise, most women can return to their prepregnancy weight in a matter of months.

Early-life obesity

The rate at which body fat is deposited is not constant throughout childhood development. There may be times when a child has too much body fat, which represents only a temporary "overshoot" of ideal body weight. At birth, body fat represents 15 percent of body weight, which is relatively low. This percentage increases to 26 percent by 6 months and then gradually decreases to about 14 to 16 percent in the 6-year-old child.

Puberty

Just before puberty, body fat increases to about 20 percent. Girls have a higher percentage of body fat than boys at any weight. Following puberty, the difference between the sexes is most significant, with the fat content of young men dropping to 13 percent and that of young women rising to 25 percent. These changes are normal and desirable and parents should not be concerned. For the vast majority of babies and young children, energy requirements are dictated by appetite. Encouraging an increase in the child's activity is far better than restricting calorie intake, at any age.

Adulthood

Both ethnic and economic differences influence the eating patterns of adults. These variations in part may reflect the diverse underlying attitudes toward eating and obesity among different ethnic groups and social strata of our society, as well as food availability and cost.

Fat variations

The graph below illustrates the remarkable variations in body fat that occur in early life. After age 1, the percentage of body fat drops as more energy is used in crawling and walking. The decline continues until early puberty. Boys lose fat in their teens, while girls retain it as part of the maturation process.

Percentage of weight as body fat (y-axis: 10–26)

Age / Months / Years: 0, 6, 1, 2, 4, 6, 8, 10, 12, 14, 16, 18, 20, 22

☐ Male   ☐ Female

HOW TO PREVENT OBESITY IN CHILDREN

The American Academy of Pediatrics recommends the following reasonable, though as yet unproved, measures to help babies and children avoid obesity.

Choose breast-feeding rather than bottle-feeding. There are physiological and psychological advantages.

Delay the introduction of solid foods until the infant is at least 4 months old (see INTRODUCTION TO SOLID FOODS on page 77).

Give food in response to hunger. Be aware of your baby's signals that indicate hunger. Encourage physical activity and exercise.

For moderately obese preadolescents or adolescents, encourage an increase in physical activity. Your doctor may recommend a balanced diet that induces a deficit of about 30 percent of the usual calorie intake, which can often be achieved by eliminating foods of high caloric density, such as fat-containing snacks.

CASE HISTORY
AN OVERWEIGHT ADOLESCENT

WHEN DYLAN GOT WARTS on his hands, his mother took him to the family doctor. But the doctor was much more concerned by Dylan's weight of 165 pounds at 5 feet 4 inches. Dylan's mother also had a serious weight problem, and the doctor realized that the boy was in danger of lifelong obesity if his eating and exercise habits were not changed.

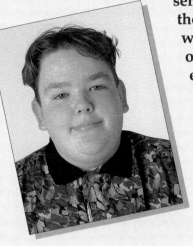

PERSONAL DETAILS
Name Dylan Richmond
Age 13
Occupation Schoolboy
Family Both parents are obese but otherwise well. Both have been advised to lose weight.

MEDICAL BACKGROUND
Dylan has had the usual childhood illnesses. Being overweight has long been a family characteristic – his mother weighs 250 pounds and his father weighs 300 pounds.

THE CONSULTATION
Questioning Dylan and his mother, the doctor learns that Dylan has a "poor appetite," eating little at mealtimes, but regularly eating hamburgers, potato chips, soda pop, and candy between meals. Even so, Dylan says he is sure that he does not eat more than his friends who are of average size. Dylan's mother tells the doctor that the only real exercise Dylan gets is in his gym class at school.

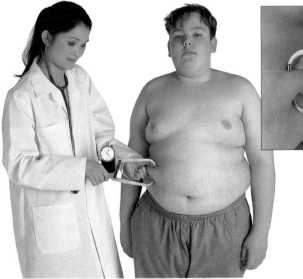

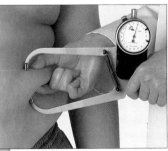

Skin-fold test
Dylan's doctor discusses his diet with him and uses calipers in a skin-fold test to confirm her suspicion that he is carrying too much fat.

THE EXAMINATION
Dylan's skin-fold thickness is several times the normal, even on his back. His skin is puffy and inflamed in areas where skin surfaces come into contact with each other, such as in his groin, between his thighs, and below his armpits. The doctor notices the beginning of a fungus infection in Dylan's groin area.

THE DIAGNOSIS
The doctor tells Dylan's mother that Dylan is experiencing the effects of OBESITY, but that they are minor compared to the risks he will run in the future if he doesn't lose weight. She says that there is little chance that Dylan will lose weight without a change in his life-style.

THE TREATMENT
The doctor, who knows it is unlikely that a low basal metabolic rate underlies Dylan's condition, is willing to accept that Dylan does not necessarily overeat all the time. She encourages Dylan to exercise much more, and he soon becomes an avid swimmer. He also walks to and from school instead of riding the bus. Dylan's mother offers him apples, air-popped popcorn, and raw vegetables as snacks and cuts down on the fat content of the family's meal. As a result, Dylan's food intake is reduced to about 1,200 kilocalories a day – about one third less than his estimated requirements.

THE OUTCOME
At age 14 Dylan joins a class organized by his junior high school and attends it twice a week for support and discussion on diet. The school also offers a special exercise program in addition to gym class. By age 16, Dylan is trim and healthy. The modifications in his life-style may help him keep the weight off as an adult.

LOSING WEIGHT

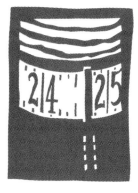

PEOPLE OF ALL AGES may feel the need to lose weight when pregnancy, overeating, or lack of exercise has led to weight gain. A weight loss program coupled with exercise offers the best chance of long-term success. It is important to choose a varied, balanced diet and set your goal for a loss of no more than 1 or 2 pounds a week. Maintaining your weight loss may require a modification of your life-style, including your eating and exercising habits.

The ideal shape
Over the centuries, our concept of the ideal figure has varied enormously. For example, the goddess Venus, portrayed below in the sixteenth-century painting by Titian, appears far fatter than today's fashion model. Although the extreme thinness fashionable in the 1960s is less popular today, some fashion images continue to cause even trim women to feel dissatisfied with their bodies. The messages that these unrealistic images convey can be depressing and can add to the social pressure people feel to lose weight.

Losing weight permanently involves much more than getting down to an optimum, safe weight. Many of us have dieted and increased the amount we exercise to achieve our target weight, only to return to our former eating and exercise habits once the scales proved we had accomplished our goal. What is important to remember is that eating too much, exercising too little, or a combination of both usually contributes to weight gain in the first place. The long-term control of weight is far more important, and far more challenging, than initial weight loss.

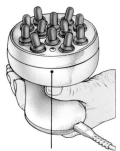

"Exercise" gimmicks
Expensive equipment and other items purported to tone the body are constantly being advertised. However, they are no substitute for diet and exercise.

Massage device

Vibrating pads

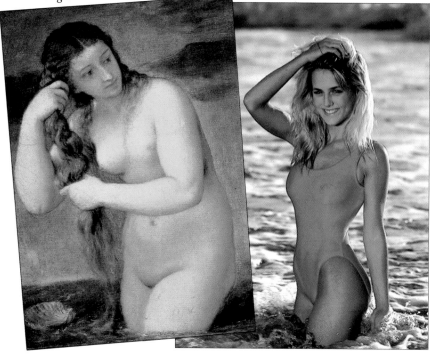

THE CHALLENGE

The challenge of losing weight permanently is reflected in the fact that the medical profession is not particularly successful in treating obesity. It is fairly easy for an obese person to lose up to 10 or 15 pounds. However, for reasons not completely understood, after the initial weight loss, many obese people reach a plateau and have real difficulty losing any more weight.

Less than 10 percent of obese patients treated by doctors are able to achieve permanent weight loss.

The greater the degree of obesity, the smaller the chances of successful weight control. It is rare for highly obese people to achieve substantial weight reduction because the factors that led to the obesity are so powerful. Tackling the problem of overeating is as difficult for some people as beating a drug addiction. Severely obese people may also find it difficult to exercise because of their size.

WEIGHT-LOSS DIETS

Losing weight involves making changes in your diet that can be maintained. Some experts believe that losing and re-gaining weight repeatedly may be more harmful than being overweight. Dieters who regain weight often end up weighing more than they did before beginning their diet.

WARNING

Before you begin any weight-loss diet or exercise regimen, consider the following:

♦ You must consult your doctor before beginning any weight-loss diet or exercise program if you are severely overweight or suffer from a medical problem such as diabetes or heart disease.

♦ Avoid any diet that drastically cuts the number of calories you ingest so that you can achieve very rapid results.

♦ Very low-calorie, liquid-formula diets should be used only on the recommendation of your doctor and only under his or her supervision.

♦ Drugs to help you lose weight should be prescription drugs recommended by your doctor and used only for short-term therapy.

♦ Restricting fluid intake during any diet is potentially dangerous; it can lead to dehydration.

♦ The use of dieting aids that contain laxatives or diuretics will not lead to significant weight loss and may damage your body.

HOW TO REDUCE YOUR CALORIE INTAKE

You can lose weight without following an extremely low-calorie diet. What is essential is that you lose weight on the kind of diet that you will continue to follow after you reach your goal. Cut out (or cut down on the serving sizes of) all the foods listed below in Group 1 and limit your daily intake of alcohol to the equivalent of 1 ounce of 80-proof whiskey (12 ounces of beer or 4 ounces of wine). Replace Group 1 foods with conservative portions of those in Groups 2 and 3. If you fail to lose weight, avoid all foods in Group 1, cut out alcohol, cut down on your helpings of the foods in Group 2, and increase intake of those in Group 3.

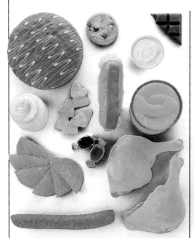

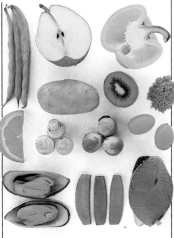

GROUP 2 (BELOW)
Meat Lean beef, lamb, and pork.
Fish Oily fish such as mackerel, herring, sardines, and salmon or tuna canned in oil.
Vegetables Legumes.
Dairy foods Eggs, 2% milk.
Others Nuts, dried fruit, bread, crackers, unsweetened cereals, pasta, rice, and polyunsaturated soft margarine and vegetable oils.

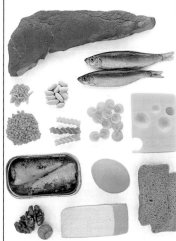

GROUP 1 (ABOVE)
Meat Meat with visible fat, bacon, duck, goose, sausage, salami, pâté, and luncheon meats.
Dairy foods Butter, whole milk, cream, mayonnaise, most cheeses, and ice cream.
Others Fried foods, potato chips, gravies or sauces, oil-containing salad dressings, sweetened cereals, cakes, cookies, candy, pastries, chocolate, jams, jellies, canned fruit in syrup, and beverages with added sugar.

GROUP 3 (ABOVE)
Meat All poultry (except duck or goose) with skin removed and liver.
Fish Nonoily fish such as cod, haddock, tuna and salmon canned in water, and shellfish.
Vegetables All vegetables, including potatoes.
Dairy foods Skim milk, plain low-fat yogurt, and low-fat cheese.
Fruit Fresh fruit and unsweetened fruit juices.
Others Bran and whole-grain pasta, bread, and cereals.

HOW SAFE ARE POPULAR WEIGHT-LOSS DIETS?

TYPE OF DIET	COMPOSITION	ADVANTAGES AND DISADVANTAGES	EFFECTIVENESS AND SAFETY
ONE-DIMENSIONAL DIETS	Diets that consist of a single food or category of foods, such as an all-fruit diet or buttermilk-only diet.	These diets have no advantages. Hunger and boredom are common. The diets often disrupt bowel function. No diet of this kind can be followed safely for more than a short time due to the dangers of nutritional deficiency.	Any weight loss achieved is usually not permanent. These diets cause losses of muscle protein and water. The weight is regained when normal eating is resumed. One-dimensional diets are not recommended.
HIGH-FIBER DIETS	Foods such as whole-grain bread, pasta, and cereals, dried peas and beans, fresh vegetables, and fresh and dried fruits, which contain complex carbohydrates and high levels of fiber.	A high-fiber diet is consistent with contemporary nutritional thinking. The bulk of high-fiber foods helps promote satiety. When eaten as part of a balanced menu, this diet provides the benefits of a high intake of dietary fiber. A disadvantage is that many people initially experience gas and indigestion. These symptoms usually disappear with time and can be avoided to some extent by adding fiber to the diet very gradually and by not eating too much fiber.	As long as the diet contains a wide variety of low-calorie foods, it is a safe way to lose weight. High-fiber foods promote weight loss because they are more filling and contain fewer calories per gram than high-fat foods.
VERY LOW-CALORIE LIQUID-FORMULA DIETS	Very low-calorie liquid formulations containing a relatively high proportion of protein. This type of diet contains protein from soy flour and low-fat milk solids and provides about 400 kilocalories per day.	These diets are of limited value. They may lead to loss of lean body tissue and may aggravate some metabolic disorders. They should be undertaken *only* under medical supervision. A number of deaths have been reported in people following this type of diet. Side effects, such as headaches, dizziness, and constipation, are common. Weight loss can be achieved but weight will return when the diet is stopped and lean body mass is restored.	These diets can be extremely dangerous. They are acceptable only for severely obese people when followed under medical supervision. The overweight person does not learn healthy eating habits and often returns to previous eating patterns.
LOW-CARBOHYDRATE, HIGH-PROTEIN DIETS	Limited amounts of high-protein foods such as red meat, eggs, and cheese. Little or no carbohydrate is consumed. Calories are not restricted.	These diets cause rapid weight loss due to loss of fluid and lean body tissue. However, because they do not reduce the amount of calories consumed, little or no body fat is lost. Furthermore, such diets can be monotonous and unpalatable, are nutritionally unbalanced, and are very high in fat. They often lead to diarrhea and fluid imbalance.	These diets are not effective. Weight loss occurs solely through loss of fluid and tissue protein. They are potentially harmful and are not recommended.
"SINFUL" DIETS	Calorie-controlled meals that include foods such as alcoholic drinks, sweet foods, and so-called junk food.	Such diets have no advantages. They do nothing to control a craving for sweet foods that inevitably persists after the diet. They consist of high-fat, high-calorie foods with low nutrient value that overweight people must avoid to stay healthy as well as to lose weight.	Such diets usually contain "empty," nutrient-poor calories that are primarily derived from nonnutritious sources. They are not recommended.
WELL-BALANCED, LOW-CALORIE DIETS	Calorie-controlled meals consisting of a wide variety of low-fat foods.	So long as these diets provide no less than 1,000 kilocalories per day and include a variety of nutrient-rich foods, they are nutritionally acceptable. Hunger may be experienced but distributing the calories so that you eat some food between meals will help.	These diets can be very effective so long as healthy eating habits are maintained after weight loss. They are highly recommended as a safe way to lose weight. Their effectiveness is enhanced with education, counseling, and regular exercise.

Can dieting be harmful?

The desire to lose weight rapidly can entice people to follow potentially harmful diets. Some people are so desperate that they are prepared to try fasting. If sustained, fasting may lead to vitamin and mineral deficiencies, anemia, acute gout, dehydration, substantial loss of lean body tissues, irregularities of heart action, and death. Fasting is occasionally used as a temporary treatment for morbidly obese people and for those who are totally immobilized, but only when it is carried out in a hospital under strict medical supervision.

Diet books are perennially popular and their commercial success is based on the promise of "effortless" weight loss. However, many fad diets are nutritionally unsound and cannot be continued for more than about 2 weeks at a time without the risk of nutritional deficiencies. Another disadvantage of such diets is that they do not teach sensible eating habits or behavior modification to help the overweight person overcome a tendency to gain weight or to overeat.

Safe dieting

The best way to achieve a safe and lasting reduction in weight is through a life-style change that includes a low-calorie diet and regular exercise. The diet should produce a weight loss of about 1 to 2 pounds a week. Most people will lose this amount on a diet of 1,200 to 1,500 kilocalories a day when accompanied by a program of increased exercise. People who are shorter, older, and immobile may need to lower their daily intake to 1,000 kilocalories.

Your goal should be to lose weight permanently to avoid repeating the damaging cycle of losing and regaining weight. It is also important to reach a safe weight that you can maintain for life, rather than aim for an unrealistically low weight that you can maintain only by periods of extreme food restriction. Regular exercise is an essential component.

HELPFUL HINTS FOR DIETERS

There are a number of ways to make the task of dieting easier. Some of these suggestions require the support and cooperation of family members, who may even enjoy participating.

SHOPPING FOR FOOD

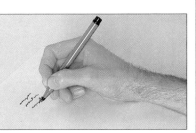

◆ Shop for food as soon as possible after a meal, when you are less likely to be hungry and tempted to buy on impulse.

◆ Make a list of the foods you plan to buy and stick to the list.

PREPARING FOOD

◆ Avoid frying your food. Try baking, broiling, poaching, roasting, microwaving, or steaming instead.

◆ When you choose to fry, stir-fry or sauté foods with a little oil or nonstick spray rather than with lots of butter, oil, or margarine.

◆ Remove all visible fat from meat and skim excess fat from stews and casseroles after preparation. The skin of poultry contains a great deal of fat and should be removed.

◆ Try to make your food interesting by using herbs and spices and low-calorie dressings.

EATING

◆ Carefully plan your meals for each day the night before or early in the morning. Plan for lower-calorie snacks (such as an apple or some unbuttered popcorn) as well as five small, well-balanced meals.

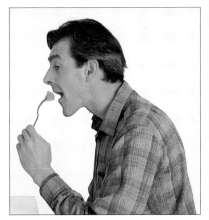

◆ Do not skip meals in the belief that it will speed your weight loss. Experience shows that it usually leads to excessive hunger and bingeing later in the day.

◆ Develop desirable eating habits. Make a decision to eat meals in the same place. Eat when sitting down at a table using a knife and fork.

◆ Cut up your food into small pieces and spread the food all over your plate. Some people find it helpful to use a smaller plate.

◆ Eat slowly, chewing each mouthful thoroughly and swallowing all the food in your mouth before putting any more on your fork.

◆ Heed your appetite cues. Avoid continuing to eat when you don't actually feel hungry.

SHAPING UP WHILE YOU LOSE WEIGHT

It is important to tone up your body while you lose weight. You can exercise at home without using any special apparatus. When performed regularly, these exercises strengthen your muscles, loosen up your joints, and gradually trim inches of fat from different parts of your body. The examples below form part of a comprehensive routine that begins with warm-up exercises and includes regular aerobic exercise, such as brisk walking, to build endurance. If you have any doubts about this type of exercise, consult your doctor. These exercises are good for toning muscles, but they can't replace walking briskly for 30 minutes every day.

Exercise 1
Stand upright with your feet about 15 inches apart and let your arms rest by your side. Bend your trunk as far as possible to your left, sliding your left hand down your leg. Hold this position. Make sure you get a good stretch. Return to an upright position and repeat ten or 12 times for each side.

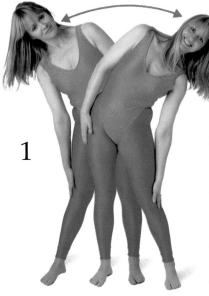

Exercise 2
Stand upright with your feet about 15 inches apart and your arms by your sides. Rotate your arms ten times forward and ten times backward. Make sure you push against an invisible force so you are not just flapping your arms but are really using your muscles. Then repeat, working up gradually to ten or 12 sets of ten.

Exercise 3
Lie on the floor on your right side, supporting your head with your right hand. Slowly raise and then lower your left leg, keeping the leg straight. Repeat ten or 12 times. Roll over and repeat. It is important to create resistance for the muscle. Don't raise the top leg higher than 12 inches or let it touch the bottom leg when lowering it. Imagine that there is a 12-inch ruler between your feet.

EXERCISE AND WEIGHT LOSS

Occasional exercise cannot reduce weight substantially because the calories burned up with a single activity are limited. With regular exercise and a controlled food intake, you will lose weight.

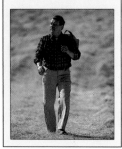

ANTIOBESITY DRUGS

The use of drug therapy to counteract obesity can be helpful, but only when combined with a program of exercise, counseling, and new eating behavior.

In the past, amphetamines were used as antiobesity drugs. These drugs act directly on the central nervous system, suppressing appetite and producing a "high" that counteracts any depression accompanying obesity and food deprivation. Many people became addicted to amphetamines, and their use is now restricted in many states. The drugs most commonly used for appetite suppression are structurally similar to amphetamines and many have similar disadvantages. They may interfere with sleep, cause depression when stopped, or cause pharmacological tolerance. Today, doctors prescribe appetite suppressants only for limited periods to help people overcome hunger and lack of willpower in the early stages of a diet.

EXTREME MEASURES

Losing weight is so difficult for many obese people that some have attempted extreme and sometimes dangerous measures. Some of these treatments have exploited the anxieties and hopes of very obese people. Others have been used as a last resort for people who are morbidly obese (either twice their ideal weight or 100 pounds over ideal weight) who have already made serious, unsuccessful attempts to lose weight by other means.

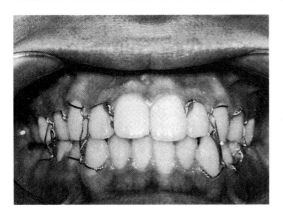

Jaw wiring
Malleable, stainless steel dental wire may be secured around several teeth near the gumline and used to hold the upper and lower teeth firmly together so that eating solid food is impossible. The procedure may lead to weight loss but not if patients have access to energy-rich, liquid nourishment, such as ice-cream sodas.

They have also been used when obesity poses an immediate, serious threat to the person's health.

Surgery

A variety of operations have been designed to interfere with the digestion and absorption of food. In the intestinal bypass operation, a loop near the beginning of the small intestine is joined to a loop near its end so that a substantial length of intestine becomes unavailable for the absorption of food. This operation became popular in the 1970s but is almost never performed today, mainly because of the risk of complications and even death.

Another operation, known as stomach bypass, involves the creation of a small pouch in the upper part of the stomach. Food is then diverted from the pouch directly into the small intestine.

Stomach stapling is an operation in which a small part of the stomach is partitioned off without altering the normal direction of food movement. This procedure has not been proven effective. In another treatment, a balloon is inflated inside the stomach to discourage overeating. The balloon method has been shown to be no better than diet alone. Complications are frequent; some are serious, even fatal.

Except for the stomach bypass, none of these surgical procedures has been successful in inducing safe and permanent weight loss except in very rare circumstances.

LIFE AFTER WEIGHT LOSS

Some dieters expect diet alone to lead to dramatic changes in their lives. When these changes fail to materialize, disappointment can set in. Many problems stem from the fact that, before the diet, food played a major part in the life of the dieter. Some people even withdraw from social activities because they are overweight. In other cases, people are unprepared for the different reactions friends have to their new bodies and feel insecure or frightened by the attention. Counseling or membership in support groups, along with exercise and new activities, can help overcome this problem.

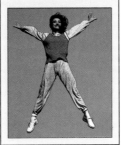

ASK YOUR DOCTOR
WEIGHT LOSS

Q Is it better for dieters to eat several small meals a day rather than one or two large ones?

A Yes, it does seem to be a good method as long as the total number of calories consumed is appropriate. Eating four or five smaller meals can also prevent between-meal hunger that can sabotage a diet. If you are trying to lose weight, you may find it easier to eat little and often. Trying to fast during the day may make you so hungry that you will be tempted to gorge yourself at dinner.

Q Would treatment with a thyroid hormone be a safe way for me to lose weight?

A No. A thyroid hormone has been used to encourage weight loss because the hormone can speed up the body's energy consumption. However, when the dose is high enough to have this effect, there is a risk of harmful side effects on your heart and other organs. In rare cases, obesity is due to underactivity of the thyroid gland. Only then is treatment with thyroid hormones appropriate.

Q I can't get rid of my extremely flabby hips and thighs. Would plastic surgery help?

A Fat deposits around the buttocks, thighs, and breasts can be sucked out using a technique known as suction lipectomy, or liposuction. However, complications can occur and large fat deposits cannot be safely removed. In addition, the reshaping is often lumpy and irregular. Fluid accumulation may develop after the operation and can lead to shock. Before you consider plastic surgery, try weight control and exercise.

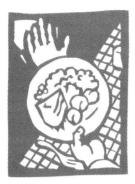

ANOREXIA NERVOSA AND BULIMIA

ANOREXIA NERVOSA is a serious condition that has caused thousands of teenage and young adult women to literally starve themselves. It can result in death. Bulimia is a closely related condition in which the sufferer repeatedly overeats and then uses quantities of laxatives or diuretics or forces herself to vomit. Treatment for both conditions is difficult and calls for expert help.

"Anorexia" simply means loss of appetite. There are few of us who have never experienced this feeling temporarily. Anorexia nervosa, on the other hand, is a psychological or behavioral disorder in which the sufferer believes she is overweight despite being dangerously thin. The person with anorexia nervosa induces starvation because of a fear that fatness will result from loss of control over diet and, perhaps, her life.

Anorexia nervosa is most common during the teenage or young adult years, though the disorder may persist, in a more subtle form, throughout life. In the US, about one in every 100 young, middle-class women suffers from some degree of anorexia nervosa. In those who are greatly concerned with their bodies, such as actresses, models, and ballet dancers, the figure is five times greater. Very often, women with this disorder are also obsessive about exercise. Five to 10 percent of patients who are treated for anorexia nervosa in a hospital later die of suicide or starvation. Anorexia infrequently affects young men.

Self image
The primary problem in anorexia nervosa is not the loss of appetite so much as the loss of a realistic perception of the size and shape of the body.

Changes in fashion
An unrealistic concept of beauty may have contributed to the increase in the incidence of anorexia nervosa in the last 30 years. Being thin has come to be identified with sexual attractiveness, and such influences may have a powerful effect on women who are deeply concerned about the way they are perceived by others.

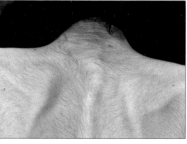

Lanugo hair
A common feature of anorexia nervosa is an excess of fine, downy hair (lanugo) over the cheeks, forearms, legs, and, as shown above, the nape of the neck.

IDENTIFYING PATTERNS

The causes of anorexia nervosa are still uncertain and elusive. In a minority of cases, it is a symptom of a serious underlying psychiatric disorder, such as depression or schizophrenia. Anorexia nervosa is almost always associated with low self-esteem. Many anorectics come from close-knit families and have a particularly intimate relationship with one parent. They are often obsessional and are usually anxious to please. Some seem unwilling to grow up.

THE EFFECTS

Anorectics may lose one third or more of their body weight. Starvation interferes with the body's biochemistry and can lead to extreme tiredness and weakness. The function of the pituitary gland is depressed, resulting in a decrease in function of the glands it controls. The production of sex hormones is upset, the most obvious result of which is the absence of menstrual periods (amenorrhea). As hypothyroidism (underfunctioning of the thyroid gland) develops, the skin becomes dry and the hair falls out.

Behavior

There are characteristic patterns of behavior that suggest a person is suffering from anorexia nervosa. Behavior becomes secretive and defensive and indicates an obvious preoccupation with food. The anorectic often feels intensely hungry but this is usually denied. She usually wears clothes that conceal the body shape.

Food and weight dominate the anorectic's thoughts. There may be constant exercising and a manipulation of relationships, which may result in broken relationships and a state of isolation. The anorectic may have difficulty sleeping and may wake early. She may resort to drugs and alcohol in an attempt to alleviate both hunger and depression.

HOW DO YOU SEE YOURSELF?

Below are five different types of figures, ranging from very thin to fat. Ask yourself which shape you most closely resemble and then ask your friends how they see you. If you think of yourself as being far heavier than your friends think you are, you may have an anorectic tendency.

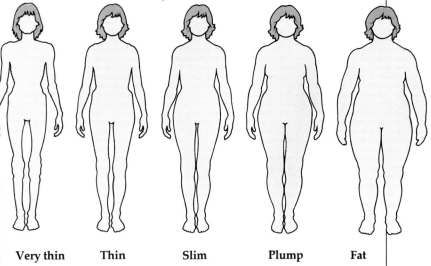

| Very thin | Thin | Slim | Plump | Fat |

THE EFFECTS OF ANOREXIA NERVOSA

Starvation interferes with the body's biochemistry and can have severe effects, some more immediately obvious than others.

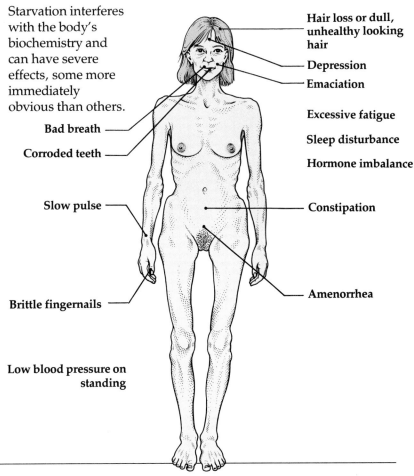

Hair loss or dull, unhealthy looking hair

Depression

Emaciation

Excessive fatigue

Sleep disturbance

Hormone imbalance

Constipation

Amenorrhea

Bad breath

Corroded teeth

Slow pulse

Brittle fingernails

Low blood pressure on standing

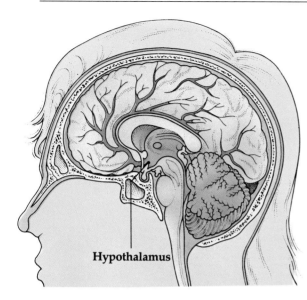

The hypothalamus
It has been suggested that anorexia nervosa is caused by a disorder in the part of the mid-brain, called the hypothalamus, that is concerned with the linkage between the emotions and the nervous system, and with such functions as hunger, thirst, and sexual activity. It seems more likely, however, that any changes that have been detected in hypothalamic function are secondary to the effects of starvation induced by psychological problems.

Hypothalamus

BULIMIA

Bulimia is often, though not always, related to anorexia nervosa. The bulimic may be of normal weight, slightly underweight, or extremely thin. She suffers from poor self-esteem and is subject to constant thoughts of eating and an irresistible craving for food, leading to recurrent episodes of extreme overeating.

A person who has bulimia suffers from a morbid fear of obesity. The result is that she feels so bad about overeating that she takes drastic measures to prevent what she sees as the natural result – gaining weight.

The bulimic forces herself to vomit by pushing her fingers down her throat and may also take doses of laxatives or diuretics. Bingeing and purging are conducted in secret and may occupy much of her time. Bulimics are also obsessive about exercise. The repeated loss of stomach acid through vomiting corrodes the teeth and causes potentially serious changes in blood acidity and potassium levels. People with bulimia are usually deeply distressed, sometimes to the point of suicide. The mortality is lower than that for anorexia nervosa because there is not the extreme wasting away of the body. Treatment is along the same lines as that given for anorexia nervosa.

DIMINISHING DIET

As a result of the conviction that she is overweight, the anorectic gradually eliminates foods from her diet until she is eating practically nothing and becomes emaciated. The condition is compounded if she exercises excessively.

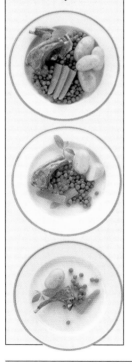

TREATMENT

Anorexia nervosa cannot be treated simply by urging or forcing the sufferer to eat. Such efforts usually prompt the anorectic to devise ingenious methods that give the appearance of eating. Expert treatment is urgently needed. Patients are often stubborn, and it is common for their behavior to cause discord between health care professionals and family members. Treatment at home is seldom successful; the anorectic usually requires an extended stay in the hospital.

A managed approach

The management of anorexia nervosa usually includes psychotherapy and a program of re-feeding. Because patients usually make every effort to circumvent treatment, strict surveillance is essential. If there is a clear indication of underlying depressive illness, drug treatment may be needed.

It is a mistake to believe that the problem has been solved once the anorectic's normal weight has been restored. Relapses are common during times of even moderate stress. About half of the young women who have been treated for anorexia nervosa need to remain under psychiatric care and counseling for months or years.

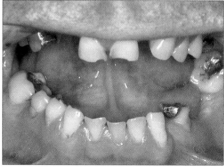

Dental damage
The bulimic's teeth are usually badly damaged by stomach acid, making them rough and sharp. This may, in turn, cause the back of the sufferer's hand to become scarred or callussed as a result of repeatedly forcing her fingers down her throat and rubbing her hand against her teeth.

CASE HISTORY
CHRONIC UNDERWEIGHT

ROBERTA IS ONE of the most promising students at the school of music she attends. Though she has missed some classes recently – and fainted one day during practice – her teachers were both surprised and concerned when she announced that she was giving up her studies. She refused to give any explanation, either to the college authorities or to her parents. After her father expressed his disappointment in her, she made an unsuccessful suicide attempt and was admitted to a hospital.

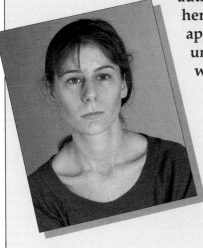

PERSONAL DETAILS
Name Roberta Rossi
Age 19
Occupation Student
Family Roberta is an only child. Her parents have always been in good health.

BACKGROUND
Roberta was moody as a child and, at one time, her parents discussed consulting a psychiatrist. Relatives always thought Roberta's moodiness was, to some degree, explained by her relationships with her parents. She has always been devoted to her father, a concert pianist, but never got along with her mother, an elegant and sophisticated woman whom Roberta sees as a rival for her father's affections. Roberta was inclined to chubbiness as an adolescent and was teased about it by both family and school friends, but especially by her father. Over the past year, Roberta has taken to wearing large, baggy clothes and appears uninterested in eating meals with the family. Her parents have assumed she is simply going through a phase of fad dieting.

THE HOSPITAL CONSULTATION
On admission to the hospital, Roberta is found to be underweight and very weak.

THE DIAGNOSIS
Roberta is suffering from ANOREXIA NERVOSA and is introduced to a psychiatrist. She is convinced that she is so fat that her father finds her repulsive. She also believes that she will not be able to fulfill her ambition of a career in music unless she loses enough weight to appear attractive onstage. She is deeply depressed.

THE TREATMENT
The psychiatrist meets with Roberta every day. Their task, along with the hospital program of feeding Roberta regularly, is to help her grow into an independent person. This is a challenge that involves discussion of Roberta's relationships with her parents. After being discharged from the hospital, Roberta has several relapses. However, both she and the psychiatrist are pleased with her progress. Eventually, Roberta moves out of her parents' house and into an apartment of her own. She also continues her studies.

THE OUTCOME
In her mid-twenties, Roberta travels to Europe for a special performance. Her success is a milestone in her process of self-discovery. She is now a successful soprano.

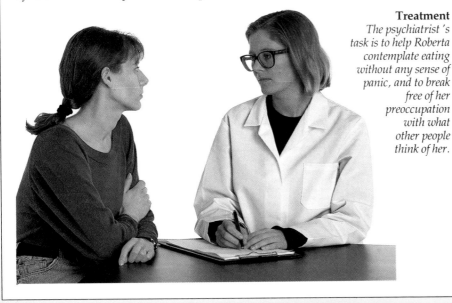

Treatment
The psychiatrist's task is to help Roberta contemplate eating without any sense of panic, and to break free of her preoccupation with what other people think of her.

CHAPTER FIVE

DIET AND DISEASE

ONCERN ABOUT the effects of our diets on our health is probably at an all-time high. Many disorders, illnesses, and symptoms have been linked to diets or substances in foods. A number of these links are stronger than others, some are weak statistical associations, and others are just pure speculation.

In this chapter, several of the primary areas of concern are discussed and recommendations are given on the selection and preparation of foods. But concern about the connection between diet and health must be kept in perspective. Foods are an integral part of our social and biological lives. They should contribute to, not detract from, health, and eating should be a pleasure. Provided we follow a few precautions, we can reduce the risk of many diet-related ills, while still eating enjoyably and well.

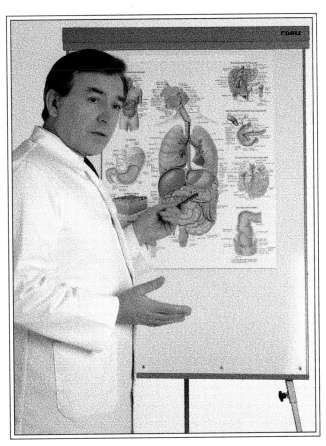

The first section of this chapter, VITAMIN AND MINERAL DEFICIENCIES, concentrates on people in high-risk groups and on the special factors that may increase the risk of deficiency. A deficiency can be precipitated by illness, by increased requirements for a particular nutrient, by a poor diet, or by a combination of any of these factors. Iron-deficiency anemia provides a classic example of this interplay.

After iron, an insufficient intake of calcium is perhaps the most significant nutritional deficiency in the US. A life-long sedentary life-style and low intake of calcium are two factors implicated in the development of the bone-thinning disorder OSTEOPOROSIS, which is discussed in the second section of this chapter.

The next two sections, DIET AND CANCER and DIET AND HEART DISEASE, provide a contrast. The dietary guidelines for preventing heart disease, which include regular exercise, less saturated fat, and more fiber in the average diet, are well known. On the other hand, there is little conclusive proof concerning the use of any dietary guidelines in the prevention of cancer.

Finally, the sections on FOOD ALLERGY AND FOOD INTOLERANCE and on FOOD POISONING examine the causes of some short-term adverse reactions to foods. Some people believe that hypersensitivity, or allergy, to certain foods is a frequent cause of uncomfortable symptoms. There is little evidence to support this notion. The incidence of food poisoning, on the other hand, may be increasing and, although few cases are serious, you may want to practice the precautions that are offered to prevent food poisoning in your home.

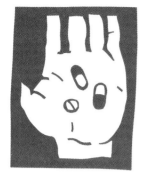

VITAMIN AND MINERAL DEFICIENCIES

MOST CLASSICAL DEFICIENCY diseases, such as scurvy, rickets, and iodine-deficiency goiter, have virtually disappeared in developed countries. However, dietary deficiencies have not been completely eliminated. Large groups of people are at risk of marginal deficiencies that produce few, if any, symptoms. Other people are sufficiently affected to suffer from mild forms of deficiency and some experience full-blown deficiency syndromes.

Digestive system disease
Diseases that increase the risk of deficiencies include celiac sprue (an intestinal disorder), inflammation of the pancreas, biliary cirrhosis (a liver disorder), and a stomach disorder that leads to malabsorption of vitamin B$_{12}$.

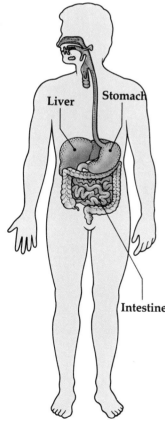

Liver   Stomach

Intestine

There are many causes and many manifestations of vitamin and mineral deficiencies. Deficiencies can arise even with an adequate diet because of a disease or illness that hampers the absorption of a micronutrient from the digestive tract, or increases its losses from the body. Deficiencies develop in some people (such as pregnant women), despite diets that would be adequate for most

Chronic illness
Vitamin and mineral deficiencies can occur as a result of chronic illness or disease, despite an adequate diet. Deficiency can usually be controlled by modifying the diet and taking supplements.

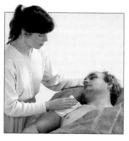

Pregnancy
Pregnancy and lactation increase a woman's nutritional requirements. Deficiencies of iron and folic acid are more likely to occur during pregnancy; intake should be monitored and supplements may be recommended by a doctor.

Poverty and famine
In many developing countries, poverty and famine are major causes of starvation and malnutrition. Vitamin A deficiency and niacin deficiency disease occur commonly in regions of impoverished countries.

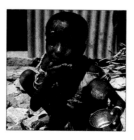

people, because they have an increased need for certain nutrients. Deficiencies develop in yet other people, such as the impoverished and alcoholics, because their diets are inadequate and their lifestyles are unhealthy. The most common deficiency disease worldwide is iron-deficiency anemia (see box at right).

DEGREES OF DEFICIENCY

The tables on pages 122 and 123 list the symptoms and effects of most full-blown vitamin and mineral deficiencies. However, marginal deficiencies are probably more common and significant because they affect the overall health of a population. Marginal deficiencies may cause vague symptoms and skin problems and can often be traced to diets that are highly restrictive or contain a high percentage of highly processed foods.

An insufficient intake of dietary calcium from birth onward, which is common, may hasten the rate at which bones become demineralized with age (see OSTEOPOROSIS on page 124).

For many trace minerals, dietary deficiencies are not recognized, simply because not enough is known about them. But that does not mean that they may not occur. In fact, surveys have found that intakes of many trace elements are lower than requirements but not so low that symptoms of deficiency develop.

IRON-DEFICIENCY ANEMIA

Iron-deficiency anemia is the most common deficiency disease in the US and worldwide. If the body contains an insufficient amount of iron, it cannot make enough of the oxygen-carrying pigment hemoglobin. Hemoglobin is needed to form red blood cells.

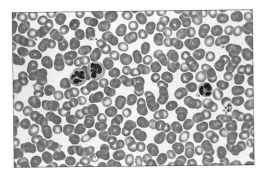

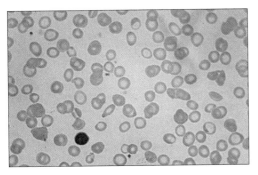

Normal and anemic blood
The photographs (taken with the aid of a microscope) compare normal blood (top) and blood from a person with iron-deficiency anemia (above). The iron-deficient person's cells are abnormally pale due to a lack of iron and hemoglobin. Because of this deficiency, their oxygen-carrying capacity is reduced.

WHAT ARE THE CAUSES?

A diet that contains an insufficient amount of iron-rich foods.

Poor absorption of iron from the digestive system.

Heavy menstrual periods, or normal menstrual periods accompanied by long-term insufficient dietary intake of iron.

Increased needs during pregnancy.

Regular loss of blood (and thus iron) in feces or urine due to diseases of the digestive or urinary tract.

WHAT ARE THE SYMPTOMS?

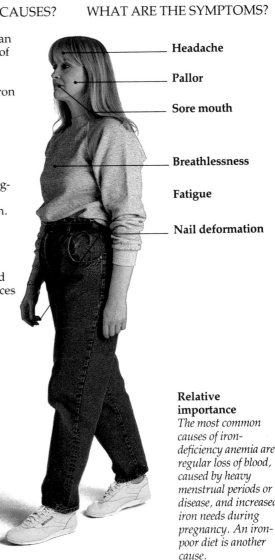

- Headache
- Pallor
- Sore mouth
- Breathlessness
- Fatigue
- Nail deformation

Relative importance
The most common causes of iron-deficiency anemia are regular loss of blood, caused by heavy menstrual periods or disease, and increased iron needs during pregnancy. An iron-poor diet is another cause.

DISEASE AND DEFICIENCY

The diseases or illnesses that can cause deficiencies are primarily those that affect the organs of digestion, absorption, or excretion. A variety of stomach, intestinal, pancreatic, and liver disorders may affect the digestion and absorption of micronutrients into the bloodstream and lead to a deficiency of vitamins such as A, B_{12}, D, E, K, and folic acid, or minerals such as calcium, iron, zinc, and magnesium. Severe vomiting and diarrhea can lead to deficiencies of potassium and magnesium. Various kidney diseases can lead to deficiency of vitamin D, calcium, potassium, and magnesium.

In all these cases, the underlying disease requires medical treatment, which may include taking vitamin or mineral supplements. Sometimes, little can be done about the underlying disorder, but good health can be maintained through attention to certain aspects of diet along with taking supplements.

Rich sources of iron
Foods rich in iron include red meat, organ meats such as liver, some green leafy vegetables, and whole-grain and enriched breads.

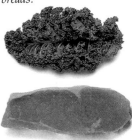

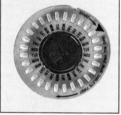

LONG-TERM USE OF MEDICATION AND ORAL CONTRACEPTIVES

Many medications can interfere with the absorption of micronutrients or with their metabolism. Some antiepilepsy drugs increase the need for vitamin D and folic acid. The use of oral contraceptives increases the need for several B vitamins, vitamin C, and vitamin E. If you are taking a long-term medication or an oral contraceptive, ask your doctor whether you need to take a supplement.

DEFICIENCY DUE TO INCREASED NEEDS

Pregnancy and lactation call for increased attention to nutritional requirements. Deficiencies of iron and folic acid are more likely to occur during this time, so dietary intake should be monitored carefully. Supplements may be recommended by your doctor (see PREGNANCY AND LACTATION on page 72).

Several circumstances, including pregnancy and lactation, may increase your need for certain nutrients. A lack of sunlight increases the need for vitamin D, and using some medications or oral contraceptives (see left) increases other requirements.

INADEQUATE DIETARY INTAKE

There are many ways in which a person's diet can be inadequate. In some cases there is a lack of food. In others, too many highly refined or processed foods (and too few fresh foods) are eaten or the number of foods eaten is too limited. Even in many developed countries, poverty is still too often the cause of an inadequate diet.

Alcoholism and drug abuse

Many chronic alcoholics eat little food and obtain a large proportion of their energy from alcohol. As a result, their intake of protein, essential minerals, and vitamins may be grossly deficient. Alcohol abuse can cause problems, such

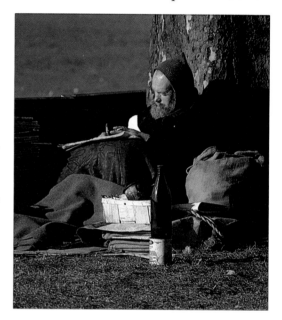

FULL-BLOWN MINERAL DEFICIENCY	SYMPTOMS OR EFFECTS
Iron deficiency	Anemia; sore mouth; nail changes
Calcium deficiency	Osteoporosis, characterized by loss of bone density and increased tendency to fractures of the spine, hip, and wrist
Chromium deficiency	Impaired ability of the body to use glucose, which raises blood glucose levels
Copper deficiency	Anemia; loss of bone mass
Iodine deficiency	Enlarged thyroid gland (i.e., goiter)
Magnesium deficiency	Tremors; muscle weakness and/or spasms
Selenium deficiency	Manifestations of deficiency not known; possible premature aging from damage to cells
Zinc deficiency	Poor growth and delayed sexual development in children; delayed wound healing; loss of appetite; increased susceptibility to infection

FULL-BLOWN VITAMIN DEFICIENCY	SYMPTOMS OR EFFECTS
Vitamin A deficiency	Night blindness; rough, dry skin; lowered resistance to infection; weak bones; absence of tooth enamel in children
Thiamine deficiency (beriberi)	Mental confusion; depression; fatigue; loss of muscle coordination; numbness and tingling of the legs; calf tenderness; weakness; fluid accumulation; sometimes heart failure
Riboflavin deficiency	Inflammation and cracking at corners of mouth; dermatitis; inflammation of the tongue
Niacin deficiency	Sore, itchy, flaky skin; diarrhea; depression; mental confusion; sore tongue
Vitamin B_6 deficiency	Anemia; dermatitis; irritability; insomnia; nervousness
Folic acid deficiency	Anemia; lowered resistance to infection
Vitamin B_{12} deficiency	Anemia; sore tongue; mouth sores; spinal cord abnormalities
Vitamin C deficiency (scurvy)	Loosening of the teeth; poor healing of wounds; bleeding into skin, joints, and gums; tender joints; susceptibility to infection
Vitamin D deficiency (rickets or osteomalacia)	Bone softening; bowing and distortion of the long bones; later, waddling gait
Vitamin E deficiency	Anemia; possible premature aging from damage to cells
Vitamin K deficiency	Bleeding tendencies

as gastrointestinal irritation or liver or pancreatic disease, that reduce the absorption of nutrients from the digestive tract or reduce their use by the body. Like chronic alcoholics, many drug abusers neglect their diet and are prone to a similar range of deficiencies.

Food fads
Food fads that involve a very low intake of food or that severely restrict the number of foods eaten can cause deficiency. For example, low protein diets may lead to niacin deficiency and total fasting can lead to thiamine deficiency as well as to mineral and protein deficiency within a relatively short time.

High intake of processed food
The refining and processing of food can cause the loss of many vitamins and minerals, only some of which are re- placed during the enrichment process. Any person whose diet consists largely of processed and refined foods can become marginally deficient in vitamins such as vitamin B_6 and vitamin E and minerals such as chromium, zinc, copper, and selenium.

DIAGNOSIS AND TREATMENT

For many nutrients, a full-blown deficiency syndrome is fairly easy to recognize and can be treated by a doctor through large doses of the vitamin or mineral. Marginal deficiencies are difficult to identify except by blood tests. However, if you suspect you have a vitamin or mineral deficiency for reasons other than illness or increased need, the reason is probably life-style, including an inadequate or unbalanced diet.

VEGETARIANISM

Vegetarians who do not eat meat or fish but do eat eggs and dairy products (lacto-ovovegetarians) are at risk only of iron deficiency. Those who eat no animal products (vegans) are at high risk of vitamin B_{12} deficiency. Unless foods are selected carefully, vegans also risk deficiencies of riboflavin (vitamin B_2), vitamin D, calcium, iron, and zinc as well as certain amino acids. A calcium supplement is also recommended.

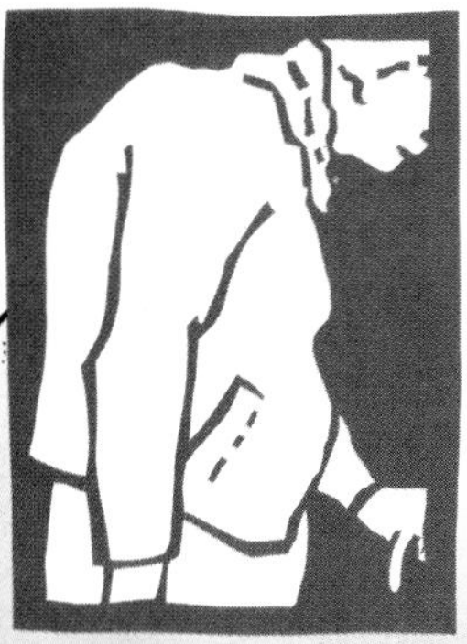

OSTEOPOROSIS

OSTEOPOROSIS IS A CONDITION in which bones become progressively less dense and weaker. It causes more than 1 million spine, hip, and wrist fractures in the US each year. Osteoporosis is generally considered to be a disease of women, but, with increasing age, men also experience loss of bone density.

NORMAL AND OSTEOPOROTIC BONE

The bone shown here is a femur, or thighbone. The left side of the cutaway shows normal, dense bone; the right side shows osteoporotic bone. The femur is one of the bones most commonly fractured because of osteoporosis.

Who is at risk?
The risk of osteoporosis increases with age. Almost everyone over 55 probably has some degree of bone loss, but women are especially at risk because the lack of estrogen after the menopause dramatically increases the rate (for a few years) at which bone density is lost.

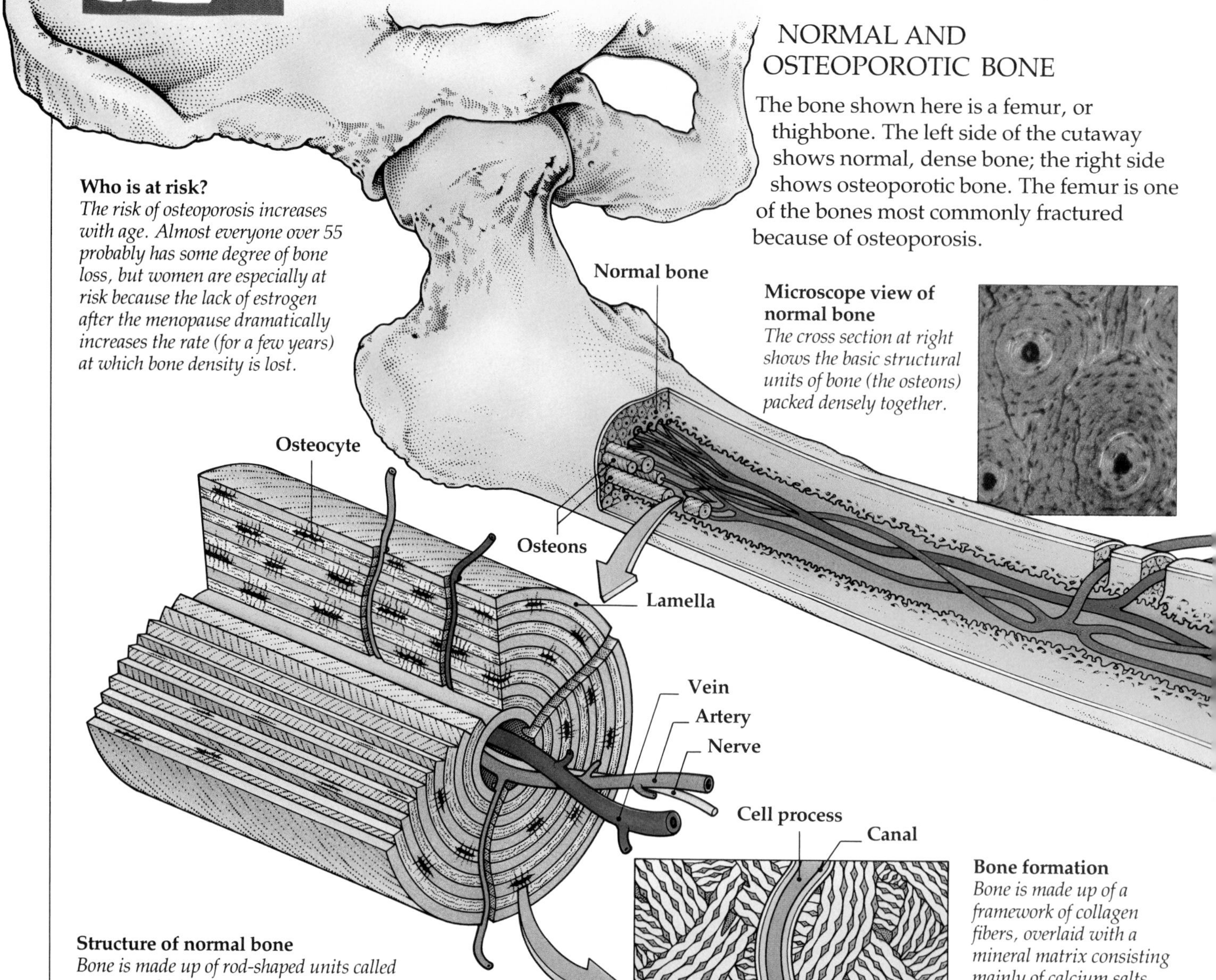

Normal bone

Microscope view of normal bone
The cross section at right shows the basic structural units of bone (the osteons) packed densely together.

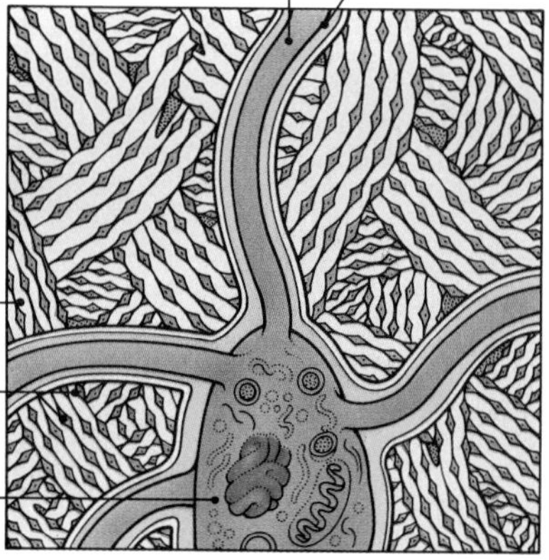

Osteocyte

Osteons

Lamella

Vein

Artery

Nerve

Cell process

Canal

Bone formation
Bone is made up of a framework of collagen fibers, overlaid with a mineral matrix consisting mainly of calcium salts. Osteocytes form the collagen and assist in the deposition of calcium salts.

Collagen

Calcium salts

Osteocyte

Structure of normal bone
Bone is made up of rod-shaped units called osteons, which consist of concentric layers. In each adjoining layer, or lamella, the collagen fibers are oriented in a different direction, contributing to bone strength. The cells trapped between the lamellae are osteocytes, which maintain bone. They are connected to each other and to the bone surface by structures that allow the interchange of calcium between bone and blood.

Microscope view of osteoporotic bone
The cross section at right of bone affected by osteoporosis shows many spaces (white areas) within the bone where protein and calcium have been reabsorbed.

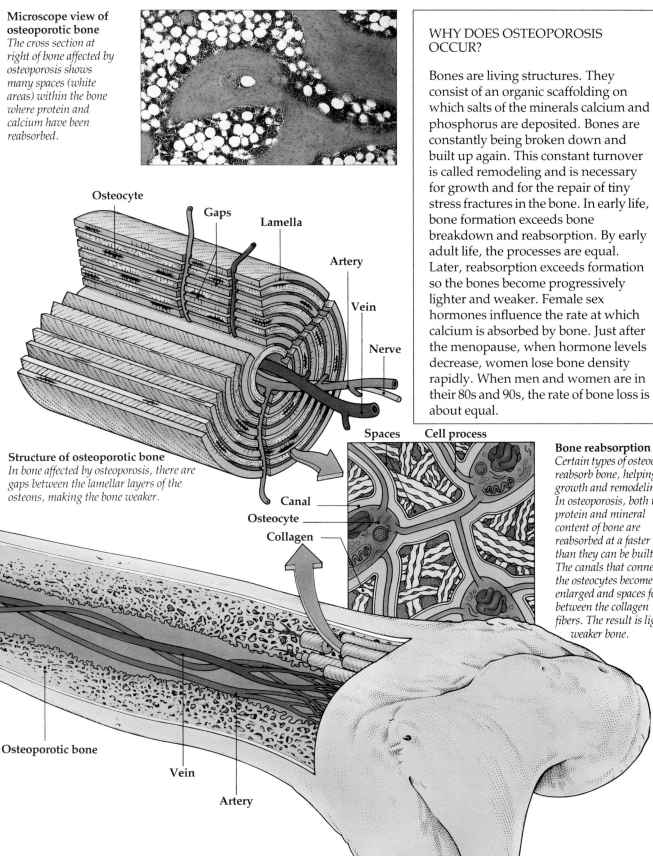

WHY DOES OSTEOPOROSIS OCCUR?

Bones are living structures. They consist of an organic scaffolding on which salts of the minerals calcium and phosphorus are deposited. Bones are constantly being broken down and built up again. This constant turnover is called remodeling and is necessary for growth and for the repair of tiny stress fractures in the bone. In early life, bone formation exceeds bone breakdown and reabsorption. By early adult life, the processes are equal. Later, reabsorption exceeds formation so the bones become progressively lighter and weaker. Female sex hormones influence the rate at which calcium is absorbed by bone. Just after the menopause, when hormone levels decrease, women lose bone density rapidly. When men and women are in their 80s and 90s, the rate of bone loss is about equal.

Structure of osteoporotic bone
In bone affected by osteoporosis, there are gaps between the lamellar layers of the osteons, making the bone weaker.

Bone reabsorption
Certain types of osteocytes reabsorb bone, helping in growth and remodeling. In osteoporosis, both the protein and mineral content of bone are reabsorbed at a faster rate than they can be built up. The canals that connect the osteocytes become enlarged and spaces form between the collagen fibers. The result is lighter, weaker bone.

EFFECTS OF OSTEOPOROSIS

The most obvious effect of osteoporosis is the increased tendency of bones to fracture in response to minimal force. In middle-aged women who have gone through the menopause, the most common fractures are of the wrist and vertebrae. In older people, both men and women, fractures of the hip are the most common injury.

People with osteoporosis may become shorter as a result of the collapse of one or more vertebrae. They may also develop a protruding curvature of the spine. In some cases, this curvature is so extreme that the head is forced down onto the chest. Crushing of a vertebra can cause muscle weakness and pain due to compression of a spinal nerve.

PREVENTION OF OSTEOPOROSIS

It is not possible to reverse osteoporosis. One of the best preventive measures is to build up the bulk of the skeleton in childhood by ensuring an adequate intake of calcium. Some doctors recommend a calcium intake of between 1,000 and 1,200 milligrams per day. The richest sources of calcium are milk and most dairy products, soybeans, broccoli, green leafy vegetables such as kale (especially collards), and canned sardines and salmon eaten with bones. Sedentary people who

HOW BONE LOSS INCREASES WITH AGE

The graph shows the percentage of bone density lost with age. Both sexes lose bone after age 30, but the rate of loss is faster in women, especially just after the menopause. Pregnancy and lactation also use up calcium reserves. Preventing osteoporosis (see below) is the best approach.

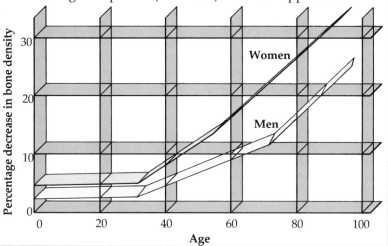

drink milk to provide calcium may want to choose low-fat milk to avoid the fat and calories.

You can strengthen your bones by doing what is called "weight-bearing" exercise regularly. The precise mechanism is not clear, but, when physical forces are applied to a bone, the osteocytes are somehow stimulated to increase their bone-building activity. Any weight-bearing exercise, such as brisk walking, done for 20 minutes three or four times a week will contribute significantly to the retention of bone density.

HORMONE REPLACEMENT THERAPY

After the menopause, the drop in estrogen levels causes rapid bone loss. The most effective means of counteracting this is by hormone replacement therapy with estrogens or a combination of estrogens and progesterone. Although it has not been established that estrogen replacement can lead to an increase in bone bulk, it can prevent further bone loss. In the US, hormone replacement therapy has halved the number of fractures caused by osteoporosis in women after the menopause.

CALCIUM-RICH FOODS

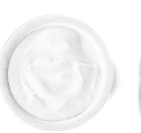

Yogurt (made from 1% milk) 8-oz container
271 mg calcium

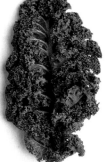

Kale 1 cup (cooked)
206 mg calcium

Tofu (soybean curd) 4 oz
146 mg calcium

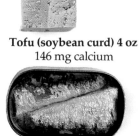

Sardines (canned, eaten with bones) 4 oz
400 mg calcium

Milk (2%) 1 cup
352 mg calcium

CASE HISTORY
PERSISTENT BACKACHE

FOR SEVERAL MONTHS, DEIRDRE has been experiencing a persistent backache, which she attributes to sitting for long periods in a deep armchair. She hasn't thought it serious enough to make an appointment with her doctor, but the pain in her back has worsened recently and she is eventually persuaded by her daughter to consult her family doctor.

PERSONAL DETAILS
Name Deirdre Keaton
Age 62
Occupation Retired saleswoman
Family She is a widow and lives alone.

MEDICAL BACKGROUND
Deirdre had a hysterectomy at 50 because of heavy uterine bleeding.

THE CONSULTATION
The doctor examines Deirdre and observes that she has a marked angulation of the middle lower part of her spine, known as kyphosis. He orders an X-ray of Deirdre's spine, as well as a series of blood tests. The doctor also asks Deirdre about her diet and exercise habits. He is not surprised to learn that she has never much liked milk, cheese, or other dairy products or made much effort to compensate for this dislike by eating other calcium-rich foods. In addition, she does not exercise – she even avoids walking to the mailbox.

THE TEST RESULTS
The X-ray shows that Deirdre's bones are much less dense than normal. Several of her vertebrae have become wedge-shaped, and there has been a recent crush fracture of two of them, which is causing the severe curvature of her spine. The results of her blood tests are normal.

THE DIAGNOSIS
The doctor tells Deirdre she has OSTEOPOROSIS. Deirdre's spinal bones have become so thin from loss of protein and calcium that their front portions have become compressed from the weight of her upper body, and two of them have collapsed.

THE TREATMENT
Deirdre is given an orthopedic support and drugs to relieve her pain. She is also given a daily calcium supplement, a small daily dose of vitamin D, and a drug containing estrogen and progesterone to take for 25 days each month. The doctor asks Deirdre to avoid heavy lifting or any other activity that might exert pressure on her bones.

THE OUTLOOK
Deirdre asks the doctor whether she should drink more milk. She also asks whether her daughter is at risk of osteoporosis. The doctor tells Deirdre that it is too late for any dietary modification to have much effect on her condition. The best she can hope for is that her condition will not deteriorate further. Deirdre is assured that there is no hereditary basis for osteoporosis. However, since her daughter is a small-boned woman, she is probably at greater risk than many women. Her daughter is advised to walk regularly and make sure she has sufficient calcium in her diet.

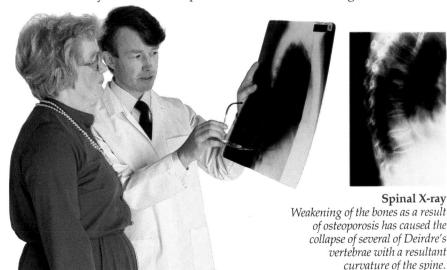

Spinal X-ray
Weakening of the bones as a result of osteoporosis has caused the collapse of several of Deirdre's vertebrae with a resultant curvature of the spine.

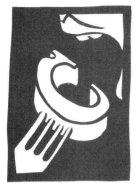

DIET AND CANCER

SOME POPULATION studies suggest that dietary factors may be responsible for as much as 35 percent of all cancers that occur in developed countries. The evidence for this claim is based primarily on studies that investigate the cancers that are common in different countries. Although no direct links have been established between dietary patterns and cancer, there are now reasons to believe that the risk of cancer might be reduced by modifying our diets.

The incidence of the main types of cancer varies greatly from one country to another. Almost every cancer that is common in the US is not as common in other countries. In addition, several cancers that are rare in the US are common in other parts of the world. Yet, in the US and Europe, the children and grandchildren of immigrants from Africa and Asia have the same patterns of cancer as Americans and Europeans who have lived their entire lives in these countries.

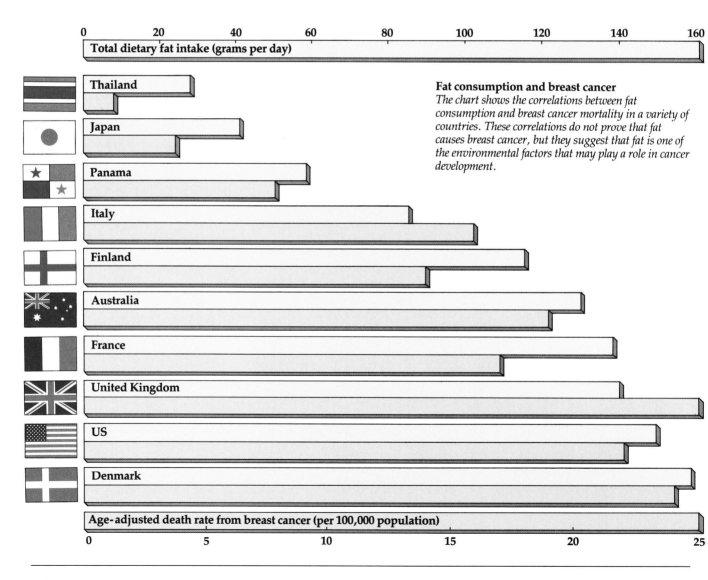

Total dietary fat intake (grams per day)

Thailand
Japan
Panama
Italy
Finland
Australia
France
United Kingdom
US
Denmark

Age-adjusted death rate from breast cancer (per 100,000 population)

Fat consumption and breast cancer
The chart shows the correlations between fat consumption and breast cancer mortality in a variety of countries. These correlations do not prove that fat causes breast cancer, but they suggest that fat is one of the environmental factors that may play a role in cancer development.

DIETARY FACTORS LINKED TO CANCER

Population surveys can only show associations between cancers and the way people live. The evidence is mainly indirect or circumstantial. The fact that a high intake of a certain factor, such as fat, is associated with an increased incidence of a certain cancer does not prove that the factor causes the cancer. There are hardly any dietary substances that have been shown to cause cancer directly.

Total fat intake
The total fat intake among the Japanese population provides close to 22 percent of all calories consumed. Americans get 36 to 41 percent of their calories from fat. The National Cancer Institute recommends that 30 percent or less of your total calories be derived from fat. This can be achieved by limiting your consumption of fatty meats, full-fat dairy products, fats, oils, and baked goods.

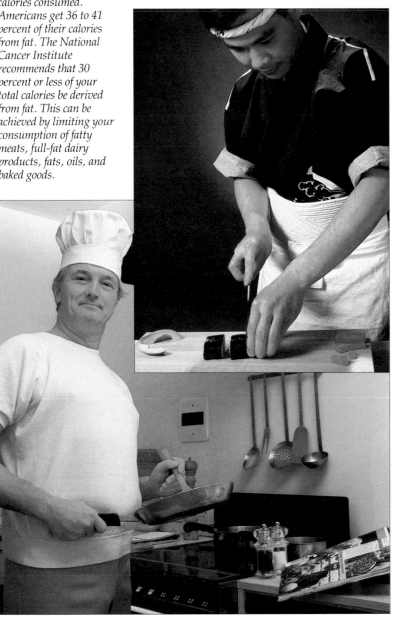

Fat

The clearest statistical association, derived from population studies, is between dietary fat and several cancers. In countries such as Japan, where the fat intake is generally very low, the rates of breast and colon cancer are low. In some countries where the dietary fat intake is high, such as the US, the rates of breast and colon cancer are high. Furthermore, children of immigrants who move from countries with different environmental factors, including a low fat consumption, to countries with a high fat consumption (such as the US) show similar patterns of breast and colon cancer to those of Americans.

The picture is complicated by the fact that diets high in fat are generally low in fiber, so there is a possibility that diets low in fiber, just as much as diets high in fat, may be causing the cancers.

If, as some of these associations suggest, the intake of dietary fat does influence the development of cancer, neither the mechanism by which it does so nor the degree to which it may play a role is known.

Obesity

Dietary fat is one factor; another is body composition. A major study, carried out by the American Cancer Society, adds to the controversy about whether obese men and women are at increased risk of cancers of the uterus, kidney, colon, and breast. Men who are more than 40 percent heavier than the optimum weight for their height have a 33 percent increased risk of dying of these cancers (excluding uterine cancer). For women who are equally obese, the risk of dying is 55 percent higher than that of women of normal weight.

These figures are difficult to interpret and statistical associations cannot prove cancer causation. However, the figures suggest another good reason to eat correctly and exercise in order to maintain your ideal body weight throughout life.

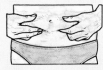
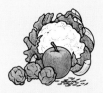
Cancer of the esophagus
This picture (above right) shows an endoscopic view of a cancer in the esophagus.

Liver cancer
This microscope picture of a liver specimen (right) reveals cancer cells.

Alcohol

A heavy alcohol intake has been firmly linked with cancers of the mouth, larynx, pharynx, esophagus, lung, stomach, liver, colon, and rectum.

Alcohol seems especially toxic when combined with excessive smoking. It appears that each agent enhances the other's damaging effect.

Nitrites, nitrates, and nitrosamines

Nitrites and nitrates are used as food additives mainly to preserve meat such as bacon or sausages. Nitrites can be oxidized to nitrates and then converted to chemicals called nitrosamines in the presence of substances found in meats. Nitrosamines are also produced by overcooking or smoking meat.

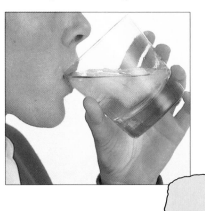

Smoking and drinking
Anyone who drinks and smokes heavily increases his or her chances of cancer of the larynx, mouth, pharynx, esophagus, lung, stomach, liver, colon, and rectum.

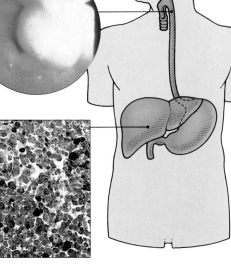

Nitrosamines are known to cause cancer in animals and are thought to be a cause of cancer in humans. Furthermore, the incidence of esophageal and stomach cancers is high in parts of the world where the consumption of smoked and nitrate-cured foods is high, such as in Japan and China. Although the role of such foods in causing human cancer is unknown, it is wise to minimize your intake until the controversy is resolved.

Benzopyrene in grilled food

Benzopyrene, a substance found on the charred surfaces of charcoal-broiled foods, has been shown to cause cancer in animals. Its effect on humans is not known. The American Cancer Society has recommended that charcoal-broiled foods be eaten only in moderation.

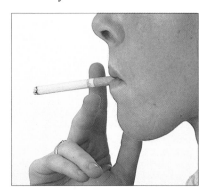

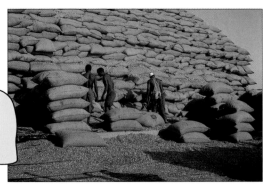

Aflatoxin
Aflatoxin is a cancer-causing poison produced by the molds Aspergillus flavus *and* Aspergillus parasiticus. *The molds grow on poorly stored and damp grains and are a common contaminant of peanuts. In parts of Africa, such as Mozambique, where control of food storage is less rigid than in developed countries, aflatoxin is a major cause of liver cancer (although infection with the hepatitis B or C virus is at least as much of a causative factor).*

SUBSTANCES THAT MAY PREVENT CANCER

Much data has been accumulated suggesting that certain dietary substances might play an active role in preventing cancer.

DIETARY FIBER

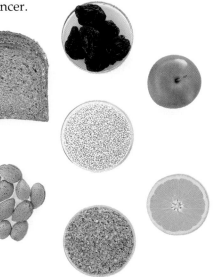

Cancer of the colon is a common cause of death in industrialized countries where, among many dietary differences, there is a high consumption of processed and refined foods with a low fiber content. Cancer of the colon is rare in many Asian and African countries where, among other differences, fiber is not refined out of the foods people eat. The role of dietary fiber in the digestive process is described on page 48.

It is speculated that by somehow changing the proportion of certain bacteria in the bowel, dietary fiber might "protect" us against cancer. Fiber also increases the fecal bulk and, therefore, may bind fecal bile acids or other possible cancer-causing substances. Fiber also shortens the transit time of the stool, thereby reducing the time that any carcinogens are in contact with the walls of the colon. However, evidence supporting the protective effects of dietary fiber is inconclusive.

VITAMIN C

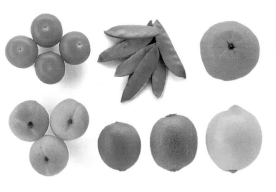

Overall, although it has not been proved that increasing your vitamin C intake can lower the incidence of cancer, there are good reasons for making sure that your vitamin C intake is at least up to the recommended daily allowance of 60 milligrams a day. Studies have shown that people whose diets contain many of the fruits and vegetables that are rich in vitamin C are less likely to get cancer, particularly cancer of the stomach and esophagus. It is not certain whether vitamin C as opposed to the other constituents of fruits and vegetables is responsible. However, vitamin C is known to inhibit the formation of some suspected cancer-causing agents.

VITAMIN A

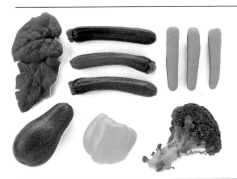

Vitamin A has been linked to a lower risk of cancer of the lung, bladder, colon, rectum, larynx, esophagus, stomach, and prostate. Though the results are not conclusive, laboratory experiments on animals and cell cultures suggest that vitamin A may operate by preventing cells from becoming transformed to a cancerous state. Good sources of vitamin A are broccoli, spinach, brussels sprouts, squash, carrots, and pumpkins, as well as apricots and peaches.

CRUCIFEROUS VEGETABLES

Cruciferous vegetables are claimed to provide some protection against cancer. Cruciferous vegetables include brussels sprouts, cabbage, broccoli, cauliflower, kohlrabi, and turnips.

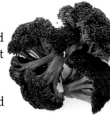
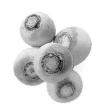
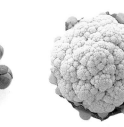

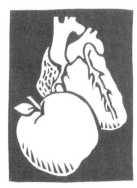

DIET AND HEART DISEASE

THERE IS NO LONGER any doubt that your diet can influence your risk of heart disease. The dramatic decline in the incidence of coronary heart disease over the past 30 years is thought to be due in large part to the conscious decision of many Americans to modify their life-styles, including a reduction in the consumption of foods known to promote atherosclerosis.

In developing countries, most diet-related heart disease is caused by malnutrition, including deficiencies in specific nutrients. Of far greater significance in developed countries, however, is the high incidence of coronary heart disease associated with a sedentary life-style, a lifelong intake of excessive calories, and a high-fat, low-fiber diet. In addition, general nutritional inadequacy (which may occur with anorexia nervosa) can lead to other heart conditions and sudden death. Deficiency of potassium and magnesium can cause irregularity of heart action and even cardiac arrest, although deficiency in these minerals is much more likely to be caused by serious disease than by inadequate diet.

SEVERE THIAMINE DEFICIENCY

Severe thiamine deficiency causes beriberi, a metabolic disorder that interferes with the function of the brain, nerves, and muscles. Thiamine is found in whole-grain products, meats (especially pork), green vegetables, potatoes, and nuts. Deficiency may occur as a consequence of starvation, alcoholism, or a very poor diet. In one form of beriberi, the heart is enlarged and its pumping capacity is reduced, resulting in congestion of blood in the veins and fluid retention.

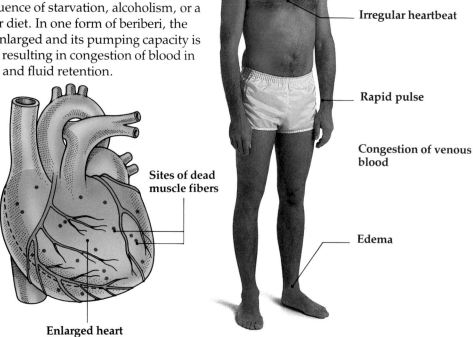

Red face and extremities

Labored breathing

Palpitations

Irregular heartbeat

Rapid pulse

Congestion of venous blood

Edema

Sites of dead muscle fibers

Enlarged heart

REDUCING BLOOD CHOLESTEROL

To lower the cholesterol in your blood, reduce the level of saturated fats in your diet to no more than 10 percent of your calorie intake. All the fats in your diet should supply no more than 30 percent of total calories. Most of your energy needs should be fulfilled by carbohydrates, especially in fiber-rich forms such as whole-grain products, vegetables, and fruit. The fiber in these foods binds with cholesterol in the bowel, helping to eliminate it. Fiber also binds bile, reducing absorption of fat and cholesterol.

TOO MUCH FAT AND YOUR HEART

In developed countries, heart disease that results from narrowing of the coronary arteries by atherosclerosis is a major health concern. The role of dietary factors, including cholesterol and saturated fat, is a subject of intensive study (see FATS AND ATHEROSCLEROSIS on page 80).

Whether a person has a high or low blood cholesterol level results from an interplay between what that person eats, how much he or she exercises, and his or her genetic characteristics (see box on HYPERLIPIDEMIA at right). A high level of cholesterol in the blood (greater than 240 milligrams per deciliter) appears to be one of the most important of the known risk factors for coronary heart disease. On the average, people with high levels have more atherosclerosis than people with low levels. A high cholesterol level usually implies high levels of low density lipoprotein cholesterol carriers in the blood (see THE TRANSPORT OF FATS IN THE BLOOD on page 32).

HYPERLIPIDEMIA

Hyperlipidemias are a group of conditions, often hereditary in origin, characterized by high levels of lipids (fats) in the blood. These conditions increase the risk of heart attack. Strict control of fat intake, especially of saturated fats, is a vital part of treatment.

DIETARY FAT AND BLOOD CHOLESTEROL

Cigarette smoking, obesity, raised blood pressure, and other factors including heredity are associated with damage to the lining of the arteries. The risk of disease is further increased by a high total blood cholesterol level. Physical fitness is receiving renewed attention because of the findings that even moderate levels of fitness protect against heart disease.

HOW BLOOD CHOLESTEROL IS REGULATED

1 All body cells incorporate cholesterol into their membranes. The cholesterol is brought into the cells by low density lipoproteins (LDLs), which pass the cholesterol to the cells through special receptors.

2 Unused cholesterol remains in the blood, where it may build up, especially if saturated fat intake is high, because saturated fat may reduce the number of receptors and prevent the cell from taking in normal amounts of cholesterol.

3 High density lipoproteins (HDLs) collect excess cholesterol from cells and transport it to the liver. From there it is oxidized to bile acids for disposal via the bile duct into the bowel.

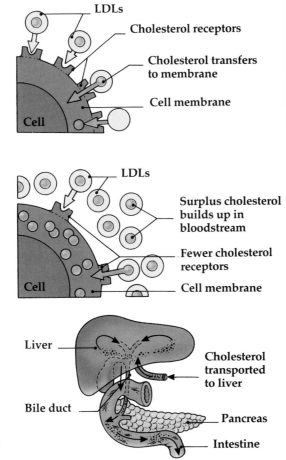

LDLs
Cholesterol receptors
Cholesterol transfers to membrane
Cell membrane
Cell

LDLs
Surplus cholesterol builds up in bloodstream
Fewer cholesterol receptors
Cell membrane
Cell

Liver
Bile duct
Cholesterol transported to liver
Pancreas
Intestine

HOW DIET CAN INFLUENCE THE RISK OF HEART DISEASE

SATURATED FATS
An excess intake of saturated fats can increase the concentration of LDLs in the blood, and suppresses the function of cholesterol receptors in the cells. Combined, these factors promote a high total blood cholesterol level.

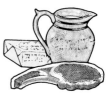

POLYUNSATURATED FATS
Provided that they replace, and are not present in addition to, saturated fats, polyunsaturated fats reduce LDL levels while leaving cell cholesterol receptors unaffected. In addition, some polyunsaturated fatty acids are believed to reduce the tendency of blood to form clots, a factor that can help prevent the occurrence of a potentially life-threatening heart attack.

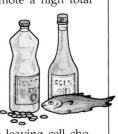

MONOUNSATURATED FATS
While high intakes of polyunsaturated fats may slightly lower levels of beneficial HDLs, monounsaturated fats reduce LDL levels without affecting HDLs. Olive oil and peanut oil are sources of monounsaturated fat. Regions where olive oil is widely used have a lower incidence of coronary heart disease than regions where saturated fats are used.

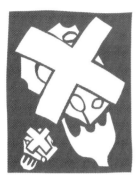

FOOD ALLERGY AND FOOD INTOLERANCE

A PERSON WHO EXPERIENCES uncomfortable symptoms after eating a certain food is not necessarily suffering from food allergy. True food allergy is a very rare condition in which some constituents of food, normally considered harmless, trigger a reaction from the immune system. More common is food intolerance, which causes transient symptoms such as abdominal distension and flatulence.

Which foods are responsible?

The foods most commonly involved in true allergy are milk, eggs, wheat, fish, shellfish, and strawberries. In rare cases, food additives have been found to cause allergy. Tartrazine, the yellow food coloring found in foods such as orange ice pops, may cause problems, especially in people who are sensitive to aspirin.

The term food allergy is incorrectly used by many people to signify any unusual reaction to a particular food, whether the reaction is brought about by immunological processes or not. In fact, reactions to food may have many causes other than allergy. The most common cause is poisoning that is the result of some form of contamination (see FOOD POISONING on page 138). In other cases, the person may lack certain digestive enzymes, or there may be a psychosomatic reaction to a food, sometimes caused by the belief that it is unclean.

ALLERGY AND THE IMMUNE SYSTEM

The function of the immune system is to protect the body from harm by microorganisms, mainly bacteria and viruses.

The immune system accomplishes this by recognizing antigens – proteins on the surfaces of the microorganisms. Cells of the immune system called B-lymphocytes produce proteins, called immunoglobulins or antibodies, that bind to proteins on the surfaces of the bacteria or viruses. This process begins the destruction of the organisms.

In the case of allergy, the immune system reacts in an inappropriate way to a substance that is normally harmless. The immune system produces a family of immunoglobulins. One sign sometimes associated with an allergy to a substance is the presence in the blood and tissue fluids of the affected person of one of these immunoglobulins – IgE. This antibody reacts to one or more allergens (substances that have no effect on people who do not have the allergy).

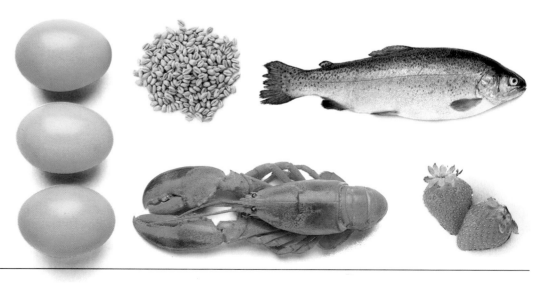

WHAT CAUSES AN ALLERGIC REACTION?

Allergy is an inappropriate reaction of the immune system to a harmless substance. In susceptible people, the reaction causes the surfaces of millions of mast cells (special cells that are especially common in the linings of the lungs and bowel) to be covered by specific immunoglobulin E (IgE) molecules, with a particular part of each IgE molecule adhering to the cell.

When allergens are introduced into the body via food or inhalation, they become bound to another part of the immuno-globulin molecules. This results in the antibody IgE molecules becoming "cross-linked." The effect is to release from the granules in the mast cells a number of powerful inflammatory reaction substances, including histamine and prostaglandins. These chemicals initiate a series of events resulting in inflammation of the affected tissues, narrowing the air passages in the lungs or provoking diarrhea. Symptoms may include dizziness, nausea, and vomiting.

THE RAST

The radio-allergosorbent test (RAST) and similar tests detect levels of IgE and thereby suggest sensitivity to certain allergens. However, IgE antibodies to food allergens are also found in a large number of people who have never experienced allergy-related symptoms, rendering direct diagnosis of allergy very uncertain. Withdrawing certain foods on the basis of results from this test does not necessarily bring relief of symptoms. For example, children who have an established milk allergy and high blood levels of IgE to milk proteins may eventually be able to tolerate milk without any change in their high antibody levels.

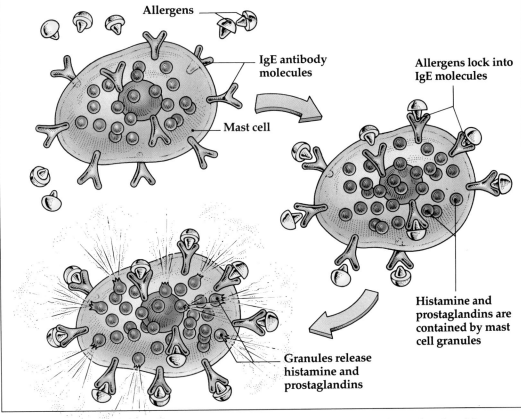

Allergens

IgE antibody molecules

Mast cell

Allergens lock into IgE molecules

Histamine and prostaglandins are contained by mast cell granules

Granules release histamine and prostaglandins

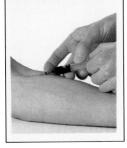

DIAGNOSING FOOD ALLERGY

Food allergy is not easily diagnosed. In patch tests, for example, samples of foods are stuck onto the skin or injected into it, and the site on the skin is monitored for inflammation or swelling. However, many different substances may cause inflammation of the skin of a patient without necessarily reflecting what will occur when the food is eaten. Books on allergy often recommend an elimination diet to identify an allergen. Certain foods are eliminated for 3 to 5 days. Foods are then added, one by one. If a food produces symptoms, it is eliminated from the diet. However, many doctors do not accept the scientific validity of these experiments because a patient's reaction may be caused by his or her expectations or by many factors other than allergy.

Double-blind trials

Double-blind trials appear to be the most reliable method of detecting allergy. They are capable of proving food allergy in only about 10 to 15 percent of persons whose history is strongly suggestive of food allergy. For the trial, a sample of the food suspected of containing the allergen is placed in one set of capsules; the other, identical capsules contain only inert material. Neither the doctor who administers the capsules nor the person who takes them knows which capsules contain the food – hence the term "double blind."

At the end of the trial, the patient is asked to decide, on the basis of any resulting symptoms, which of the capsules he or she had a reaction to. True allergy will consistently produce symptoms only when the capsules with food in them are swallowed.

FOOD INTOLERANCE

Nonallergic food intolerance is at least 10 times more common than food allergy. The problem may be the result of an enzyme deficiency rather than an immune response. Symptoms associated with food intolerance include headache, depression, flatulence, or diarrhea.

Diagnosing food intolerance

Elimination diets are also used to identify the foods causing food intolerance. However, as stated earlier, a person who associates certain symptoms with certain foods is highly likely to develop those symptoms when he or she knowingly eats the food. Nevertheless, doctors supervising elimination diets have reported the disappearance of many symptoms when certain foods were eliminated from the diet.

FOOD INTOLERANCE AND ENZYME DEFICIENCY

Food intolerance is frequently associated with a deficiency of a specific enzyme in the body. The enzyme may be a part of the digestive system, such as lactase and pancreatic lipase (shown right). Insufficient amounts of lactase result in an intolerance to the lactose (milk sugar) in milk, while a deficiency in pancreatic lipase causes intolerance to dietary fats.

Deficiencies can occur in enzymes elsewhere in the body. For example, a deficiency in monoamine oxidases – enzymes that break down highly active substances called amines – may result in migraine after the ingestion of certain foods.

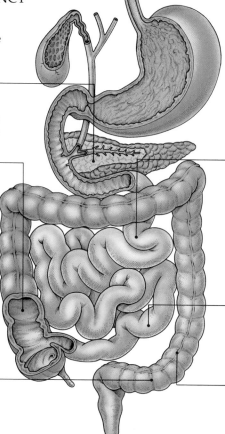

LIPASE DEFICIENCY

Cause
Inflammation of the pancreas affects production of the enzyme lipase.

Effect
Fats in the diet pass undigested into the lower part of the bowel.

Result
Bacteria partially ferment the fats, producing stools that are bulky, greasy, lightweight, and foul-smelling.

LACTASE DEFICIENCY

Cause
In most people, the cells that produce lactase become deficient after weaning. In adults, temporary deficiency may occur after intestinal flu.

Effect
Lactose in milk ordinarily splits into glucose and galactose. Without lactase it does not split, but passes undigested into the lower part of the bowel.

Result
Bacteria ferment undigested lactose, causing symptoms of gas and diarrhea.

CASE HISTORY
AN EMBARRASSING BOWEL DISORDER

ROGER IS A QUIET, **sensitive man who, for some months now, has been embarrassed by excessive gas, loud noises in his abdomen, and persistent diarrhea that has necessitated frequent visits to the washroom. He teaches at a junior high school and is becoming more and more concerned about going to work each morning.**

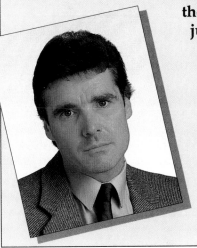

PERSONAL DETAILS
Name Roger Klein
Age 33
Occupation Teacher
Family Roger is unmarried and lives alone.

MEDICAL BACKGROUND
As an infant, Roger suffered from many colds and sore throats. Until he was 2 years old, he had frequent bouts of mild diarrhea.

THE CONSULTATION
Roger tells his doctor about the gas and rumbling, adding that for several months his abdomen has felt painfully full and distended.

THE DOCTOR'S IMPRESSION
The doctor learns that Roger is also suffering from bloating and watery diarrhea. Roger's appetite is not affected, his diet is normal, and aside from the intestinal symptoms he is generally healthy. Palpating Roger's abdomen, the doctor finds no bowel tenderness. During the rest of the examination he finds no indication of appendicitis, diverticulitis, or inflammatory bowel disease. The doctor is concerned by the amount of intestinal gas and suspects that something in Roger's diet is being acted on by bacteria in the lower part of the bowel.

FURTHER INVESTIGATION
The doctor arranges a lactose tolerance test. Roger is given 50 grams of milk sugar (lactose) and blood samples are taken at intervals. The doctor finds that the level of sugar in Roger's blood rises very little, suggesting that the lactose is not being broken down into the monosaccharides that are easily absorbed by the body. Within 2 hours, Roger is suffering more than ever.

THE DIAGNOSIS
The doctor explains that lactose is normally broken down by lactase, an enzyme produced by cells in the lining of the small intestine. If there is an enzyme deficiency, an intolerance to lactose may result. The failure to split the lactose molecule in food causes defective absorption and, when the sugar passes into the large intestine, it attracts water from the body and is fermented by bacteria, resulting in diarrhea and gas.

A fecal examination reveals that Roger is infested with the intestinal protozoon parasite *Giardia lamblia* and a blood test shows antibodies to this organism. The parasite damages the cells that produce lactase, just as Roger's frequent colds had in infancy. The doctor diagnoses an inherent tendency to LACTASE DEFICIENCY, precipitated into the full-blown syndrome by GIARDIASIS.

THE TREATMENT
Roger is given an antiprotozoal drug to eliminate the parasite. He is also asked to reduce his milk intake. Within 2 weeks the abdominal rumbling has ceased, his bowel movements are normal, and he is no longer troubled by excess gas.

Lactose tablets

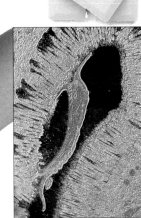

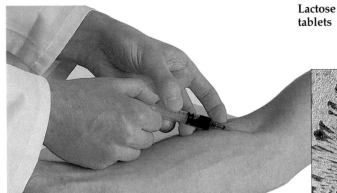

Cause and effect
By giving Roger lactose tablets and then taking blood samples, the doctor confirms his suspicion of lactase deficiency. The problem was caused by Giardia lamblia *(right), a parasite found in Roger's feces.*

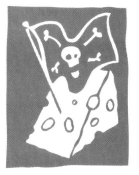

FOOD POISONING

F OOD POISONING is an illness brought on by eating food or drinking water that is contaminated with bacteria, viruses, molds, chemicals, or toxins. Typically, it causes abdominal cramps, nausea, vomiting, and diarrhea. Most people suffer at least one attack at some time in their lives. A contaminated food can look, taste, and smell fine.

Food poisoning is a rather common occurrence. It is difficult to know exactly how many cases there are each year, because the true incidence of food poisoning is thought to be greater than the number of cases reported. This may in part be due to the brief duration of the illness, which many people resolve at home without seeing their doctor.

THE INCIDENCE

In 1985, for example, there were 65,347 reported cases of food poisoning in the US caused by salmonella bacteria, 40 percent of which occurred in children under age 5. In the same year, there were 17,057 reported cases of food poisoning

The spread of disease
There are several ways in which the organisms responsible for food poisoning can be spread. Contamination of food can take one of three routes.

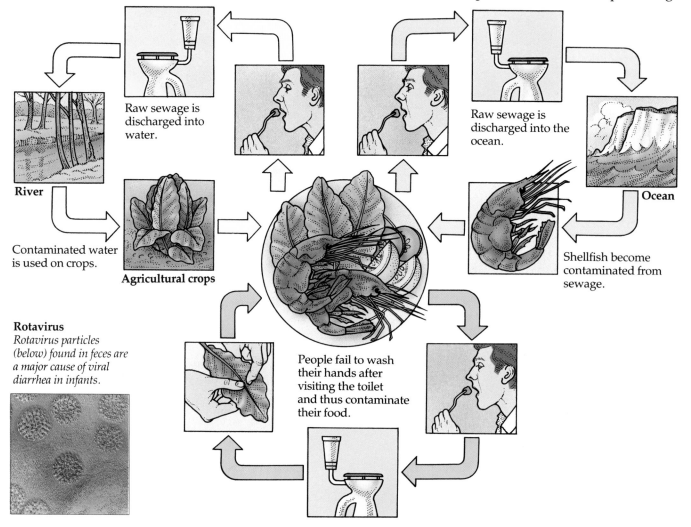

River

Contaminated water is used on crops.

Raw sewage is discharged into water.

Agricultural crops

Raw sewage is discharged into the ocean.

Ocean

Shellfish become contaminated from sewage.

People fail to wash their hands after visiting the toilet and thus contaminate their food.

Rotavirus
Rotavirus particles (below) found in feces are a major cause of viral diarrhea in infants.

caused by shigella bacteria. Yet the Centers for Disease Control estimates that more than 2 million Americans suffer from a bout of salmonella food poisoning and approximately 300,000 have a shigella infection each year.

It is not difficult to explain this discrepancy. When food poisoning affects just one person, causing only mild symptoms from which he or she recovers quickly, the attack is attributed to a "bug" and never reported to a doctor. It is only when several people become ill after eating the same food that food poisoning is suspected and an investigation is made.

Salmonella

Salmonella, of which there are hundreds of different strains, is the bacterium most commonly responsible for food poisoning. Contaminated poultry and eggs are the main sources. Salmonella can be spread to almost any food from feces, either by flies or by an infected person not washing his or her hands after using the toilet. If food is allowed to be exposed to the air for prolonged periods at warm temperatures, small amounts of salmonella can multiply into numbers that will produce toxic symptoms.

Listeria monocytogenes

This bacterium is found naturally in vegetation, soil, and water and is present in many foods, notably soft and blue-veined cheeses, pâté, and chicken. The very young, the elderly, pregnant women, and people with a weakened immune system are particularly vulnerable.

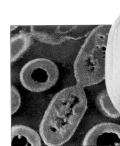

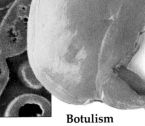

Botulism

This is a rare, serious, and often fatal type of food poisoning caused by a Clostridium botulinum *toxin.*

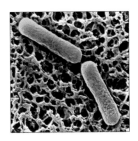

Campylobacter fetus

Campylobacter fetus *is another common bacterium of the digestive tract. Poisoning is usually caused by contaminated chicken, beef, water, or milk.*

HOW MANY BACTERIA?

Under the right conditions, bacteria will double in number every 20 minutes. This means that a single bacterium can multiply into 512 bacteria in just 3 hours.

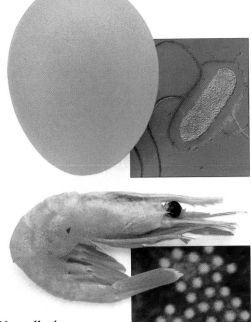

Norwalk virus

The Norwalk virus is a common contaminant of shellfish. It particularly affects adults.

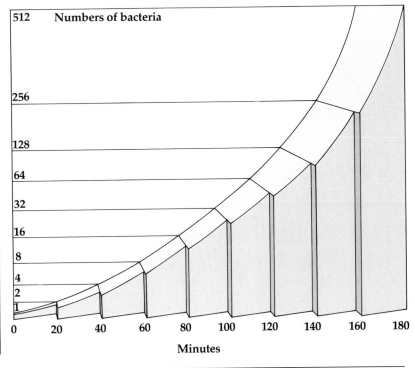

Numbers of bacteria / Minutes

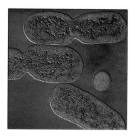

Shigella
Infection with these bacteria is usually the result of fecal contamination of food, either from hands or from flies.

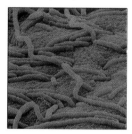

Bacillus cereus
This spore-forming bacterium is found in uncooked rice. Spores survive boiling and, if leftovers are not refrigerated, toxins are produced.

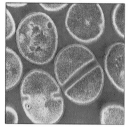

Staphylococci
Staphylococci are found in infected skin. An infected person may contaminate food, where the bacteria multiply and release toxins.

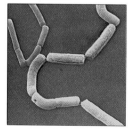

Clostridium perfringens
This bacterium occurs in contaminated meat, poultry, or vegetables.

How serious is it?

Most cases of food poisoning are not serious. The symptoms usually subside as quickly and as dramatically as they came on, and full recovery generally occurs within a few days. People who are more vulnerable to the effects of food poisoning (and may therefore not recover so quickly) are the very young, the elderly, and those with any serious, long-term illness that has weakened their natural defenses.

The most dangerous forms of food poisoning are *Listeria* poisoning and botulism. *Listeria* poisoning is particularly hazardous to pregnant women (in whom it can cause stillbirth or miscarriage) and to newborns (in whom it can cause meningitis). Botulism damages the nervous system and can be fatal.

WHAT ARE THE SYMPTOMS?

The symptoms of food poisoning depend on which bacterium, toxin, virus, or other factor has caused the illness. The symptoms vary in severity, depending on how heavily the food was contaminated. They include, most commonly, nausea, vomiting, diarrhea, and abdominal cramps. Food poisoning may also cause headaches, fever, chills, rash, and muscular pains. The time between eating contaminated food and the onset of symptoms can range from a few minutes to several days (see table below).

CAUSE	SYMPTOMS	ONSET
Bacillus cereus	Diarrhea and vomiting	2 to 14 hours
Clostridium botulinum (botulism)	Difficulty speaking, blurred vision, and paralysis	12 to 36 hours
Campylobacter fetus	Diarrhea	2 to 6 days
Clostridium perfringens	Abdominal cramps	6 to 12 hours
Chemical poisoning	Diarrhea and vomiting	Within 30 minutes
Listeria monocytogenes	Influenzalike illness	7 to 30 days
Salmonella organisms	Diarrhea and vomiting	8 to 48 hours
Shigella organisms	Diarrhea and abdominal cramps	2 to 3 days
Staphylococcal organisms	Vomiting	1 to 6 hours
Viruses	Diarrhea and vomiting	12 to 48 hours

WHAT SHOULD YOU DO?

If you suspect that you have a severe case of food poisoning, see your doctor as soon as possible so that tests can be performed to establish the likely cause and source, and the public health department can be notified.

Milder cases can be treated at home. It is important to drink plenty of clear fluids so that you don't become dehydrated. You may be advised to take a special salt and sugar rehydration mixture, available from pharmacies, until you have stopped feeling sick.

Don't eat any solid food or drink milk until your diarrhea and vomiting have stopped. Then begin with a light meal, such as dry toast and clear soup.

CHECK ON TEMPERATURES

Most bacteria thrive in warm temperatures of between 50° and 120°F (10° and 49°C). Use a refrigerator thermometer to make sure your refrigerator temperature is 41°F (5°C) or below, and your freezer temperature is 0°F (−18°C) or below. Also, use a meat thermometer to ensure that meat is cooked to at least 180°F (82°C). Do not allow foods to sit at room temperature for extended periods.

160°F and above (71°C and above) **Bacteria die**
50°F to 120°F (10°C to 49°C) **Bacteria thrive**
41°F and below (5°C and below) **Safe storage**

HYGIENE

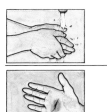

♦ Wash your hands after using the toilet. Wash your hands before handling food and after handling raw meat.

♦ Do not handle food without plastic gloves if you have an infected cut or sore on your hand.

♦ Use a clean tasting utensil each time you sample food during the cooking process.

♦ Clean all utensils and cutting boards thoroughly with soap and very hot water.

♦ Launder your kitchen dishcloths, towels, aprons, and pot holders regularly.

♦ Throw out the garbage in your kitchen and in your bathrooms every day.

WHAT CAN YOUR DOCTOR DO?

Your doctor's diagnosis will usually be suggested by the types of food that you have eaten and the length of time it took for symptoms to develop. Most cases of food poisoning clear up with rest and liquids. However, if tests are required, they may involve sending samples of vomit, feces, and leftover food to the laboratory for examination under a microscope and for culture.

Antibiotics may be prescribed for some types of food poisoning. If you have become severely dehydrated, you may be admitted to a hospital for intravenous fluid replacement.

If a toxin or a chemical poison is suspected, you will probably be sent to the emergency room to have your stomach pumped to wash out any residual poison. In the case of botulism, you will be given a special antitoxin to try to minimize damage to your nervous system.

GOLDEN RULES IN THE KITCHEN

Remember three key rules: keep hot food hot, keep cold food cold, keep all food clean. Following these rules and using common sense will protect you from most food poisoning. Here are some more tips:
♦ Do not store any food where it may touch raw meat.
♦ After you prepare raw meat wash the preparation surface thoroughly.
♦ Do not use food from containers that leak, bulge, or are damaged.
♦ Wash fresh fruits and vegetables in cold, running water.

PARASITIC INFECTIONS

Certain animal parasites can contaminate food or water. Amebiasis and giardiasis are caused by protozoan (single-celled) animal parasites. Infestation leads to persistent diarrhea that requires drug treatment. Both are usually acquired abroad but can be contracted in the US. Trichinosis is caused by a worm in improperly cooked meat. After an incubation period of between 1 and 2 weeks, it can cause diarrhea and vomiting with headaches, fever, and muscle tenderness.

ASK YOUR DOCTOR FOOD POISONING

Q What should I do about the food in my freezer if there is a loss of electric power?

A Keep the freezer door closed. Don't peek to check on the food. A fully loaded freezer will keep food frozen for 2 days. A half-full freezer will keep food frozen for 1 day. Meats that still contain ice crystals or have been maintained at 41°F (5°C) or below for less than 2 days may be refrozen.

Q I have a dog and three cats and I worry about my children picking up germs or worms from them. What can I do to minimize the risk?

A Around 50 percent of cats and dogs – particularly puppies and kittens – excrete *Campylobacter* bacteria and *Toxoplasma* parasites in their feces. Worms such as *Toxocara* are also common. The animals' coats can become tainted and can pass on the contaminants to humans, especially to children who pet the animals and then put their hands in their mouths. It is important to keep your pets' food and water bowls separate from your kitchen utensils. Do not allow pets to lick from your dinner plates. Don't feed pets raw meat and poultry, which could infect them and, in turn, you.

Q I've heard that barbecuing is not a very safe way of cooking. What is the problem with barbecuing?

A The main problem is that it is easy to blacken the outside of meat without fully cooking the inside. It is important to make sure meat is cooked to 180°F (82°C). One way to ensure that meat, such as chicken, is cooked through is to cook it in a microwave before placing it on the grill.

INDEX

Page numbers in *italics* refer to illustrations and captions.

Photograph sources:
Barnabys Picture Library **86** (bottom left)
Alan Cash **130** (center right)
Bruce Coleman **88** (bottom left); **88** (bottom center); **88** (bottom right)
Colorific Photo Library **84** (left); **120** (bottom)
Robert Harding **12** (left); **122** (right)
Holt Studios Ltd **53** (bottom)
The Image Bank **2** (bottom right); **9**; **14** (bottom); **57**; **84** (right); **112** (bottom); **113** (bottom)
R.P. Juniper **113** (top)
Living Technology **130** (center left)
National Dairy Council **53** (center)
National Medical Slide Bank, UK **12** (right); **114** (right); **116** (right); **121** (bottom)
The Photographers' Library **11** (left)

Pictor International **97**; **129** (bottom); **129** (top)
Picturepoint Ltd **108** (bottom left)
Science Photo Library **2** (bottom left); **45** (top left); **45** (top right); **45** (bottom right); **66** (bottom right); **71** (bottom left); **71** (center right); **104** (center); **105**; **121** (top); **124** (center right); **125** (top); **127** (bottom right); **130** (bottom left)
Transworld Features **108** (bottom right); **114** (left)
Tony Stone Worldwide **7**; **21**; and **front cover**
John Watney Photo Library **104** (bottom)
C. James Webb **48** (center right)
Zefa Picture Library **61** (bottom left)

Index:
Susan Bosanko

Illustrators:
Paul Bailey
Russell Barnet
Karen Cochrane
David Fathers
Tony Graham
Andrew Green
Gilly Newman
Lydia Umney
John Woodcock

Commissioned photography:
Steve Bartholomew
Susanna Price
Clive Streeter
Airbrushing:
Imago
Janos Marffy
Retouching:
Roy Flooks

Reader's Digest Fund for the Blind is publisher of the Large-Type Edition of *Reader's Digest*. For subscription information about this magazine, please contact Reader's Digest Fund for the Blind, Inc., Dept. 250, Pleasantville, N.Y. 10570.